I0415031

Collateral Damage

A Patient, a New Procedure,
and the Learning Curve

Collateral Damage

by

Dan Walter

ISBN-13: 978-1456471606
ISBN-10: 1456471600

Copyright © 2011 Dan Walter

All Rights Reserved

www.collateral-damage.net

Introduction

THIS IS THE STORY of what happened to my wife, Pam, at Johns Hopkins Hospital in March of 2002. I write this story for Pam because she endured so much unnecessary suffering at Hopkins, and because—beyond the scars and the physical insult and injury she suffered— there lingers something just as hurtful: Hopkins' refusal to acknowledge that they failed in their duty to care for her. Johns Hopkins is a great institution, revered by many, and when an icon of American 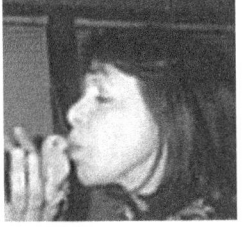 medicine casts you aside as non-creditable goods, it hurts, especially when you were a nurse and had believed yourself to be among colleagues.

By denying responsibility, Johns Hopkins Medicine is telling Pam that the ordeal she underwent doesn't matter, and that her life means nothing.

In an article called "The Malpractice Lottery," Rick Kidwell, who was Hopkins' head litigator at the time, said that "once people see juries making the big awards to patients, the number of claims often increases. It's like the theory of sharks being attracted to blood in the water." This telling of Pam's story is not about money. If there is blood in the water, it is Pam's blood, and it is not her doing. She doesn't feel like she won the lottery; quite the reverse. For the most part, "Collateral Damage" is a story about the failure of an institution rather than of its people. My aim is to accurately portray what happened to my wife at Johns Hopkins Medicine without detracting from the skill, kindness and compassion of the majority of the people who work there. Although she can no longer work, Pam is a nurse by trade, from a family of nurses, and I know how great is the capacity for caring in the medical profession.

My larger purpose in writing this book is to prove to Pam that she does matter, and to tell her that despite what the leadership of "America's Best Hospital" says, her life is important—and her story is important—and it deserves to be honestly told.

Chapter One

A Mitral Valve, Flapping in the Breeze

"Doctors love to patronize and dominate. Their arrogance and indifference to the philosophy of informed consent is widely known. Surprisingly, most residents and doctors in teaching public hospitals tacitly endorse such reservations against information sharing. To most of them getting informed consent is a needless nuisance, to be delegated to a raw resident whose sole responsibility is to get the patient's signature on the dotted line."

– Issues in Medical Ethics

JOHNS HOPKINS MEDICINE has a long tradition of prioritizing patients, and striving for the bottom rung are the anonymous poor. If, for example, you catch a bullet on a Baltimore street corner, or your mother presents you at the ER as a feverish welfare child, then it's open season for the medical students, well meaning as they may be. They can practice on you because if their actions result in an adverse outcome—which is to say that if you are mangled or killed—nobody will question said outcome, precisely because... you are a nobody.

At the other end of the spectrum are wealthy and prominent patients, important people who get treated by doctors who have already learned what not to do from the mistakes inflicted upon the lower classes.

My wife landed somewhere in the middle.

We had somehow gotten the impression that she was going to be treated by the best doctor at "The Best Hospital in America," and felt ourselves very fortunate.

Hugh Calkins, MD was to maneuver tiny wires around in my wife's heart and burn scar tissue in the wall of the atrium to stop 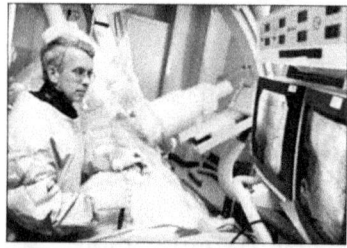 atrial fibrillation. The job required someone with a cool head and a keen eye, and Hugh Grosvenor Calkins, MD, FACC, FAHA, FHRS, Professor of Medicine, Director of the Electrophysiology Lab at Johns Hopkins University School of Medicine—and graduate of Harvard Medical School—assured us that he had done plenty of these procedures, and, he said, "experience counts."

So we knew we were in the best of hands. What we didn't know is that Professor Calkins—according to what he later told colleagues—follows the practice at most teaching hospitals wherein "the attending shows up to be there during the burn."

At Hopkins, then, the patient is etherised upon a table and wheeled into the lab, where a student of the procedure stands masked and ready for some on-the-job training. Under bright white light, the rookie's blue latex fingertips feel their way up the smooth soft skin of the exposed groin, goose bumps because it's cold in the room, pressing and probing and picking a spot, the point of a large-bore needle pressing into the skin until it punctures and there is blood.

The trainee inserts the catheter sheath into the vein, snaking it up into the pumping heart. The fine wire catheter is then fed into the sheath.

And here is where you would expect the experienced attending physician to take over because it is a very tricky business to navigate a thin wire around in a beating heart guided by cloudy X-ray imagery, even if you know what you're doing.

But since he only "shows up to be there during the burn," Hugh Calkins was presumably relaxing with colleagues down in the doctor's lounge or out selling TASER guns while a young cardiology trainee by the name of Richard Wu—whom we'd never met—was sweating out a decision in the lab.

He had a stranger laid out before him and a new type of catheter in his hand. The business end of this particular catheter uncoils to form a circle as it emerges from its sheath, which is positioned in the upper left chamber of the heart. When you turn the catheter handle clockwise, the tip uncoils into the left atrium and is ready to be put to use. Richard Wu turned the catheter handle counter-clockwise, transforming the instrument into a corkscrew, which he drove through the mitral valve of my 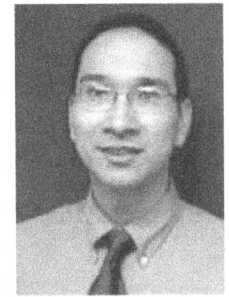 wife's heart. He didn't realize it until later, when he tried to place the catheter elsewhere in the heart and he could not do it. It was stuck.

"Only the first 50% of the circular portion of the catheter tip could be withdrawn into the sheath and pulsatile motion could be appreciated" is what they wrote in Pam's chart.

Pulsatile motion.

They were pulling on the catheter wire, trying to cajole it off a snag, but it was tugging right back, like they'd hooked a five-pound bass. A nurse notes that the "patient is waking and moving around with chest pain @ 7/10."

By that time, Hugh Calkins had shown up. He scrubbed in.

Taking hold of the controls, feeling in his fingertips the tautness of the wire and the pulsing tug of muscle from deep in Pam's heart, he turned the catheter knob this way and that, but he could not pull it free.

To see what he could see, he called for a stat echocardiogram; and yes, the distal portion of a Biosense Webster Lasso catheter was stuck deep in the wrong chamber of Pam's heart, entwined in the intricate webbing of the mitral valve muscles.

He had to stop the procedure, had to think a minute and try to figure out what to do. He called his EP lab partner, Ron Berger, who was in the middle of supervising an ablation training session down the hall. Berger surveyed the situation, scrubbed in, and gave it a try.

He turned the knob. He pulled and pushed and twisted. No good.

Stuck.

And the situation turned out to be like Chinese finger cuffs, where the more you tried to free it, the more it became entangled—and they tried for the better part of an hour, making a bad situation that much worse before finally giving up and calling for expert colleague Jeff Brinker, who studied the echo film while an assistant helped him scrub in.

The catheter was snarled tight in there all right, and Brinker saw only one chance to avoid the humiliating spectacle of having to wheel down to the surgeons a patient from the EP lab with a catheter wire tangled in her heart.

You might get lucky with a good hard yank. It says on the box to not do that because it is very likely to cause a lot of damage, but he figured it was worth a try.

As if he'd been handed a stubborn bottle of ketchup to open, Jeff Brinker gripped the control knob tightly between thumb and forefinger and prepared to apply force. Feeling the twitching pulse of Pam's life vibrating through the wire, Brinker settled into the rhythm.

One, two, *three...*

According to the record, the catheter is "suddenly free." It could not have been a good feeling for Dr. Jeff Brinker when he felt the line go slack. The sudden loss of tension meant that something had ripped or broken. Something wasn't right.

"Blood pressure dropping," someone said.

"Patient is waking and moving around reports chest pain 7 out of 10."

Eager to see what exactly had happened, the team called for another echo and was soon watching a little black & white X-ray movie, which provided Hugh Calkins with some vivid imagery for his report.

Essentially, Jeff Brinker had just ripped Pam's mitral valve muscles out by the roots, and just as the warning on the catheter package had foretold, a lot of damage had been done. Calkins wrote that most of Pam's mitral valve was "flapping in the breeze and had prolapsed into the atrium."

So there stands Jeff Brinker, staring at the bits of bloody flesh clinging to the tip of the catheter, and there's my wife, feeling intense pain and moaning through the oxygen mask they strapped over her face. She is half awake, her blood pressure is plummeting and she's in danger of dying from acute congestive heart failure.

Such a situation at a different hospital would have meant immediate open-heart surgery.

But Johns Hopkins is a teaching hospital and the patient was apparently expendable because Calkins decided to continue with the ablation procedure. He needed this one on the books, so they kept going, working the wires for almost an hour more, mapping and burning and burning again, while her breathing became more ragged and her pulse slowed and her health and vitality seeped slowly away.

Finally, with the procedure formally accomplished—so as to qualify as a success for purposes of the study Calkins was conducting—all the catheters were pulled from Pam's body and she was wheeled down to the Critical Care Unit for observation,

where surgeons informed the bumbling cardiology staff that she
would die if they didn't immediately perform open-heart surgery to
repair her valve.

After the botched ablation, I waited in Pam's room in the CCU
for her to wake up. She was not conscious because of the extra
painkillers and anesthetics she'd finally been given. One of the
drugs is called Versed, as in VERsatile SEDative, which is not a
pain medicine, but a hypnotic relaxation drug that renders patients
unaware and prevents them from remembering anything. It is one
of the more common date rape drugs.

Pam would have no knowledge of what had just happened to
her, wouldn't remember a thing. The most recent image in her
mind would be the reassuring look her daughter's eyes.

My God, I thought. When she wakes up, how am I going to tell
her?

From behind the curtain, Hugh Calkins appeared, and with him
was a young man in wrinkled and sweat-soaked scrubs, a young
man I'd never seen before who was shaking like a French soldier.
Calkins said to me that he was sorry. Really sorry.

The mapping catheter had gotten sucked into the mitral valve
because he—Hugh Calkins—had turned momentarily away from
the procedure to switch catheter sheaths.

He said he had turned his back for a second and it got away
from him, saying it like someone who had lost a child a in crowd.
"It was only for a second," he said. "It just got away from me."

At that point I felt kind of badly for him.

"It's O.K. Doc," I said.

I couldn't figure out why the young guy with him was so
shaken up, but I had more important things to worry about, like
how to break certain news to Pam once the Versed wore off.

The afternoon vigil turned out to be one of many to come over
the next three and a half weeks as Pam came close to death time
and again at Johns Hopkins, finally emerging scarred and disabled,

her life changed forever. The venerable Johns Hopkins refused to take responsibility, on the grounds that my wife should have known all along how risky the procedure was. She should have known—and she would have known—had Hugh Calkins told us what his real agenda was and what he really thought about the procedure, which is something I found out on the Internet years later.

And despite the best efforts of the administration at Johns Hopkins, I eventually found out about Richard Wu, this physician whose initial contact with my wife came as he was moving his hand up the inside of her thigh, taking his first tentative steps up what Calkins would later describe as the steep and rocky learning curve of a procedure with unprecedented risk.

They say the saying at med school is "see one, do one, teach one" and by the time I caught up with him, Wu was teaching the procedure at the University of Texas Southwestern Medical Center at Dallas. I called him for an explanation. He was very emotional, very defensive. He told me that he had spent a lot of time carefully discussing the risks and benefits of the procedure with Pam and me.

Then he denied having been involved in the "complication."

But as he struggled to alter past events for my benefit, there was something that Richard Wu didn't know—which was that his mentor and accomplice had already let the truth slip out.

Chapter 2

VERITAS

“The fact that this procedure was performed at a
teaching hospital is not relevant... Patients admitted to
teaching hospitals do not understand that they will be
subject to trial and error by students and any general
consent to be used as a teaching prop is probably itself
illegal... Finally, the responsibility to assure that a
fully informed consent has been obtained falls squarely
on the physician doing the procedure...”

– Ward Ethics

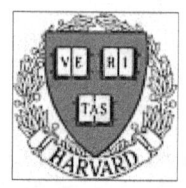 THE MOTTO AT HARVARD, where
Hugh Calkins attended medical school, is *Veritas*.
As a serious and determined young physician in
the making, the future Professor of Medicine at
Johns Hopkins University (*Veritas Vos Liberabit*),
must have laid eyes on that motto thousands of times—so often
that he probably stopped seeing it after a while, its impact literally
diminished by degrees until it became intellectual white noise.
What likely did stick in his mind was the Statue of Three Lies. It is
a bronze sculpture of a founding father type looking out over
Harvard Yard.

One supposes it to be a likeness and tribute to the founder of all
things Crimson, John Harvard, since that is what is engraved on
the base of the statue: John Harvard, Founder, 1638. But the
nickname has it right. Each finely chiseled line
is a lie.

The likeness is not that of John Harvard,
who did not found the institution, which was
not founded in 1638. And it would have been
there in Harvard Yard at the Statue of Three
Lies where, as is the custom, a young Hugh Grosvenor Calkins
rubbed his hand on the bogus founder's shoe for luck before
turning to take on the world.

The narrative presented by Johns Hopkins via their muscular stable of attorneys goes something like this: Pam Walter grabbed Hugh Calkins by the lapels one day in 2001 and demanded a catheter ablation procedure because she could no longer stand living with atrial fibrillation and she wanted something done short of open heart surgery.

Hugh Calkins discouraged the idea, telling Pam that he didn't know if the procedure was safe. Hell, he didn't even know if it worked, and he warned her that catheter ablation for atrial fibrillation is the most dangerous EP procedure there is. He advised her that contrary to public perception, going to Hopkins for a procedure is akin to going to the barber college for a haircut —except you don't get the discount. And since it is a teaching hospital, he would hand the job to a trainee whom she would never meet and who would be using new and unfamiliar instruments.

According to Hopkins, the myriad conflicts of interest that infest the country's largest health sciences research center were fully disclosed. Calkins told her that what he was really doing was conducting a de facto medical trial. He was experimenting with two new ablation techniques and testing out a couple of new mapping catheters.

He was trying out the new Biosense Webster Lasso mapping catheter and the new basket catheter put out by EP Technologies, a division of Boston Scientific. He was also collecting performance data on the new Chilli ablation catheter for Cardiac Pathways.

Calkins disclosed that he was getting paid in one way or another by all of these outfits, but Johnson & Johnson was kicking down the salary for the fellow who would be working on her, so her body would probably be used to experiment with the Lasso catheter. He told Pam that she should be aware that William R. Brody, president of the university, was on the board of directors for a major medical device manufacturer that did business with the hospital. Pam Walter was made aware in no uncertain terms that these procedures are sort of like shakeout cruises for new medical devices and their operators.

Cardiologists had done this procedure on dogs and now they were going to try it out on people, and Pam would be one of the first customers for the trial-and-error phase.

Calkins was not running any of this by the FDA, which he considered to be irrelevant, nor was he running any of it by the Hopkins Internal Review Board, because they'd rather not know what went on in his EP Lab.

Being a prudent physician, whose paramount concern is the safety of the patient, Hugh Calkins would have urged Pam to give more thought to medication and to not undergo pulmonary vein isolation using catheter ablation because, truth be told, he really didn't know what he was doing just yet.

That's what he would be using Pam for, as a body upon which to test new theories, assess new technologies and train new cardiologists.

According to Hopkins, the patient had been given all the information she needed to make a fully informed decision.

Chapter 3
The Procedure: Ready for Prime Time

"Few Decisions bespeak greater trust and confidence than the decision of the patient to proceed with surgery. Implicit in that decision is a willingness of the patient to put his life or her life in the hands of a known and trusted medical doctor... the doctor who, without the consent of the patient, permits another surgeon to operate violates not only a fundamental tenet of the medical profession, but also a legal obligation."

— Supreme Court of New Jersey

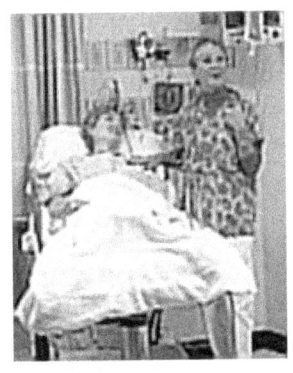

IN THE BROCHURES about Catheter Ablation for Atrial Fibrillation at Johns Hopkins, there are pictures of smiling, grateful patients sitting up shortly after the procedure, watching television or entertaining visitors. Looks like you don't even have to spend the night at the hospital: "When patients are done with their procedure, they need to lie quietly for several hours, but can eat and drink, and, as shown here, enjoy a good television show. All recovery rooms come with television sets. Nurses check on patients routinely to make sure they have everything they need."

A regular day at the spa.

A 1999 Hopkins press release touting catheter ablation for arrhythmias other than Afib announces "the first comprehensive, multi-center study of the techniques [sic] effectiveness is now complete. It was led by Johns Hopkins director of electrophysiology Dr. Hugh Calkins." The procedure is represented as being proven and painless, safe and effective:

Study Affirms Value Of Non-Surgical Treatment For Arrhythmia

BALTIMORE, MD Jan. 18, 1999 – A widely used nonsurgical treatment for rapid heart rhythms is safe and beneficial for both children and adults, according to results of a national study led by Johns Hopkins physicians...

A doctor guides a catheter with an electrode on its tip to the source of the problem. It then fires a painless burst of energy, ending the electrical misfires. Problem solved.

"This is the first large multicentre study to suggest that radiofrequency catheter ablation is safe and effective therapy and that it can now be considered as an alternative to drug therapy in the treatment of certain cardiac arrhythmias," said Hugh Calkins, M.D., lead author of the study and director of electrophysiology at Hopkins.

"The technology has now advanced to the point at which we can do the procedure on an outpatient basis, curing patients within a matter of hours and sending them home the same day," Calkins said.

Problem solved. Same day.

The basic findings of the study were that catheter ablation is in fact a safe and effective procedure. Patients are cured in a matter of hours.

Overall, on more than a thousand patients, it was successful 95 percent of the time, had a six percent recurrence rate, and a three percent incidence of complications. Equally rosy scenarios are painted on a Hopkins website about the Afib procedure, entitled *Finally a Way to get Rid of Afib,* published in 2003.

It tells the literally heart warming story of one David Erdman, a rugged outdoorsman who was "sure he had climbed his last mountain" because his Afib was getting worse.

After an episode of heart palpitations during a recent hiking expedition caused him to fall by the trail side, Erdman was sure he was going to die:

> But Erdman's cardiologist felt differently. He'd heard that electrophysiologist Hugh Calkins was offering a new technique to treat Afib at Hopkins and encouraged his patient to give it a try. Calkins would thread a catheter from Erdman's leg up to his heart and, using a high-energy probe, burn the tissue that was causing the problem...
>
> Results have been encouraging. The ablation has been able to cure 80 percent of the patients Calkins has treated for intermittent Afib and 50 percent of those with chronic Afib. The secret to success, Calkins says, is knowing how to use MRI and a special catheter-shaped like a branding iron and armed with some 20 electrodes-to zero-in on the disruptive tissues in the four pulmonary veins.
>
> "Target the active pulmonary vein and the success rate jumps to 90 percent," he says, "The procedure is ready for prime-time. Physicians and their patients should know about it."

Essentially, Hugh Calkins was claiming to the public that he had a cure for atrial fibrillation in 2003. The last word from Hopkins is that "Erdman hasn't experienced Afib in a year and currently is planning a six-day backpacking trip to Mt. Whitney in California's High Sierras."

What is proclaimed to the public while trolling for customers is different from what is written in medical journals. Pam and I had been living in Brochure Land, where the outlook is always sunny, bright and confident.

But in the professional journals, which patients don't read because they trust their physicians, the landscape is much more grim, and strewn with complications and bad outcomes.

This professional dispatch from Hugh Calkins was written in 2005, three years after he nearly killed my wife:

> "...there has never been a procedure in the field of electrophysiology with such a high complication rate. There have been more than a handful of deaths from this procedure, and as more and more people start doing it and are on that learning curve, it could be a bit of a mess."

Indeed.

I stole a book from one of the Hopkins libraries, Matt Groening's "Work is Hell." I had, of course, intended to return it when I was done, but now I'm keeping it.

I was down there in the library to try to learn about Pam's medical situation. I wanted to be able to ask the doctors intelligent questions.

I looked up mitral valve and learned that it is so named because it resembles a bishop's mitre hat. It is essentially a check valve, which allows blood to flow through in only one direction.

When there is negative pressure the valve closes—unless of course one of your mitral valve leaflets has been ripped from its base and is "flapping in the breeze" and "prolapsed in to the atrium."

Then you have what Hugh Calkins described as "complete flail," which means the valve is blown wide open, resulting in "severe regurgitation," so that blood that should be pumping out to the aorta is being sucked back into the atrium.

The echo report reads: "severe mitral regurgitation with a highly mobile mass attached to the posterior leaflet of the mitral valve consistent with ruptured papillary muscle."

"Flapping in the breeze." Indeed it had been, like a semi-detached flag in a hurricane, all during the time that Calkins or Richard Wu or someone else was hurriedly working to finish up and complete the procedure before Pam died so they could keep the stats up for the study that was in progress.

I spent a lot of time down there in the library, and the more I read about the procedure, the more I began to realize that this doctor did not know what he was doing, that he had not been telling us the truth, and that America's Best Hospital was a dangerous place to be.

Chapter 4
Delay would be Dangerous, Potentially Catastrophic

AS FOR PAM'S CHANCES of surviving her early contribution to the learning curve as she lay unconscious that day in the CCU, it may have been his instinct to soften the blow, or it may be he didn't know any better, but Calkins said that the mitral valve repair could wait until morning. He and Richard Wu, still a-tremble, then slipped away. If it could wait until morning, I thought, maybe things weren't all that bad.

Surgeons, however, were not so sanguine. I could hear the hushed and urgent voices in the hall. A chart note tells it:

"CCU Attending... Plan: Urgent MV repair/replacement... I believe delay would be dangerous, potentially catastrophic..."

I was being told with increasing frequency that while this surgery was not an emergency as such—and Pam was at liberty to refuse—she would die if she elected to forgo the pleasure.

So now the plan was this: as soon as Pam came around, expecting me to hand her some street clothes so she could come home, I was to instead hand her a clipboard with a consent form to sign, authorizing surgeons to crack open her chest so they could repair her freshly eviscerated heart.

"And we can't wait too long," advised a fatherly surgeon, "If we don't do this right away, she will not make it." "OK," says I, a bit stunned, wondering why, if it's a life and death situation, they don't just go ahead and fix it. Like right now.

But they needed her signature. They couldn't act to save her life until she signed a copy of the very same form which had, hours earlier, given them license to endanger her life.

How did we get here?

As I was pondering this, Calkins slid the curtain back and stood at the end of Pam's bed, Richard Wu behind him like a shadow. Calkins had a question for me. Did I know of any reason why Pam shouldn't take blood thinners on a daily basis? Did she have bleeding stomach ulcers or anything like that? Was it OK for her to be on blood thinners permanently?

Because there was a chance maybe that they couldn't fix the valve, they might have to replace it and, ah... you wouldn't want a mechanical heart valve in you without taking blood thinners, you know, because of clotting and all... Of course, there are pig valves, porcine valves...

I chose my words carefully because, after all, I hadn't been to medical school. "She doesn't have bleeding stomach ulcers as far as I know... So, I guess I wouldn't let that stop me..." Then I remembered a visit to the ER some months back when she'd been sick and had thrown up some blood, but they scoped her and found nothing and the situation seemed to resolve itself. But Professor Calkins and his mysterious minion had disappeared, leaving the curtain wide open.

He's asking me. I suppose that was the first time I started looking around and wondering if this was really the famous Johns Hopkins Hospital – America's Best Hospital. And as it turns out, if Calkins had bothered to read Pam's chart, he'd have seen a note in his own handwriting that "she has a history of GI bleeding."

I especially needed things to go well because, smooth assurances notwithstanding, Pam was a bit apprehensive about undergoing this procedure—or any procedure for that matter.

She was a cardiology nurse and knew full well that stuff happens, which is why we wanted her in the most experienced hands.

I encouraged the decision to go to Hopkins. "It's the best hospital in the country" I said, "and we only live an hour away." How lucky can you be?

She told me a joke on the drive up there:

A frog phones the Psychic Hotline and is told, "You are going to meet a beautiful young girl who will want to know everything about you." The frog gets excited at this prospect and says to the psychic, "That's great! Will I meet her at a party or what?"

"No, not at a party," said the psychic. "Next semester in her biology class."

The experience begins when you drive up to the front of the hospital, a large and impressive structure upon a hill. The classic dome of the original Victorian building dominates an otherwise forlorn east Baltimore landscape.

The valet staff is crisp, cordial and efficient. Gleaming doors part as you enter a large atrium, like walking into a grand train station. Before you have a chance to feel lost, a smiling greeter appears to sort you and set you on the right path.

Then, before you know it, you have surrendered your autonomy and are sitting in a wheelchair with a medical staffer propelling you down a corridor paneled on both sides with large reproduction covers of US News & World Report, confirming over and over that you have been safely delivered into healing hands at the best medical facility in existence.

For Pam, that ride took place about eight hours ago, and as I held her hand in the CCU and mulled over how exactly to break the news to her when she woke up that things… well, things hadn't gone precisely according to plan, various surgeons were sidling up to the bed, looking things over, checking monitors, reading strips.

Just checking, they'd say… just checking.

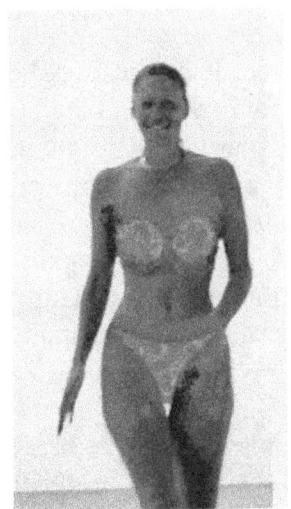

When I met Pam she was in really terrific shape—and even more so about six or seven years earlier when she went to Jackson Memorial Hospital in Miami for an EP study to be performed by Dr. Richard Luceri. The way Pam recounts the story, it was a theater-in-the-round sort of deal: "I was naked on the gurney except for a tiny hand towel covering my breasts and one laid between my legs. Young men in white coats began lining up behind the glass walls of the theater."

Pamorama.

Pam said "two EP fellows entered the lab and began probing my groin, slowly moving their fingers, pressing this way and that. Then they went and got the big needle and they started sticking me, looking for the femoral vein."

She said "They were at it for 20 minutes and I was crying when Luceri came into the room." Luceri whisked the boys aside and stuck her once and true and finally the catheter was properly placed. The whole episode had the feel of a skin flick, Pam said.

"I was taught as a nurse that before I ever walked into a patient's room, I was to always respect and protect a patient's privacy, modesty and dignity, and that's what I did in my 20 years of nursing," Pam told me.

"It didn't matter who was around or not around. It didn't matter if I was alone in the room bathing the patient. I protected their privacy. I protected their dignity and their modesty, it didn't matter if they were conscious or not," she said.

"It didn't matter if they were demented or delusional or anything else... I saw it as a basic human right, and one that I would expect for myself. Yes, and that is how I would expect to be treated, but it is not how I have been treated."

This story is loaded with coincidences: I met Pam because she was a nurse in the ICU where my father took four months to die.

He died from a series of medical mishaps that started with an overlooked staph infection picked up from a previous hospital visit —an infection that eventually destroyed one of the valves of his heart. Ron Peterson is the Chief Executive of Johns Hopkins Medicine, and Dr. Peter Pronovost is the Hopkins Safety Guru. Both of their fathers died in hospitals because people made mistakes.

Professor Luceri, who would later join Hugh Calkins in the TASER stun gun business, found nothing amiss with my wife's physiology and dismissed her symptoms with that catchall diagnosis used by male doctors who find themselves at a loss: female hysteria.

Pam's condition was real. The quest for relief from her cardiac symptoms eventually led her to Johns Hopkins and a decision that nearly cost her life, a decision based on misplaced trust in a deceptive and dangerous doctor.

Her symptoms were never as severe as those of Dave Erdman, the fabled mountain climber whose legend lives on in the High Sierras.

But alas, Pam's local cardiologist (who would later join the staff at Hopkins) had heard about the work Hugh Calkins was doing at his lab in Baltimore.

So I took my wife to Johns Hopkins.

And now here in her hospital bed she opened her eyes and she smiled and I brushed her hair from her forehead.

"Listen," I said.

Chapter 5
Drag and Burn

IN 1987, A HEART SURGEON named James Cox discovered a new use for the scalpel. If a person with Afib was having heart surgery for some other condition, Cox could make a series of small incisions in the heart while he had it right there in his hand. The scar tissue emerged in the pattern of a maze, which blocked the path of errant electrical impulses and controlled atrial fibrillation. It has proven to be a reasonably safe and effective procedure.

It wasn't long before cardiologists were trying to accomplish the same thing, using a hot-tipped catheter wire instead of a scalpel to make scars on the inside the heart, thus avoiding open-heart surgery. The idea soon caught on and competition in the medical device industry began driving research into development of a catheter-based version of the maze procedure as the cure for atrial fibrillation. The market would be very lucrative for such a cure, with more than 2.2 million Americans afflicted and the number likely to double in the next 10 years.

Relatively simple forms of cardiac ablation were already being widely performed to treat less complicated heart rhythm problems. For a condition called atrial flutter, for example, burning a small, focused scar in a certain spot in the right atrium with a catheter could usually get the job done.

Atrial fibrillation was another matter entirely. Afib researchers believed early on that they needed to create continuous lines of scar tissue, or maybe even a series of scars, in the upper right chamber of the heart.

They adapted existing technology by pushing a hot-tipped catheter to the far side of the heart and then dragging it back like a lit cigarette. The "drag and burn" was about as graceful and precise as trying to fish your keys out of a locked car with a coat hanger. It was a crude and blunt method and a far cry from the tiny surgical incisions expertly placed by the steady hand of Dr. James Cox.

Regardless of how they went about doing it, dragging a hot wire around in the top right chamber of the heart had never really proven to lessen anyone's atrial fibrillation troubles. Although sketchy preliminary data was interpreted as promising, most researchers—including Hugh Calkins—believed that success and professional glory lay in obliterating certain sections of tissue in the left atrium, the far chamber, but that was a much trickier prospect and still a long way off.

In the meantime, they had to start somewhere, and more than anything else, the right atrium was accessible.

Ultimately, the consensus on the drag and burn method was that while it had shown some potential, it was too crude to be set loose on the populace—which is really saying something.

In the journals, Calkins emerged as an early true believer in catheter ablation for atrial fibrillation. One way or another, he was going to nail down the cure within the next few years.

In an editorial headlined *Progress Continues in the Quest to Cure Atrial Fibrillation with Catheter Ablation Techniques*, he rallied for better tools.

"Although the feasibility of curing atrial fibrillation with catheter ablation has been demonstrated using standard techniques, the procedure is extremely time consuming and associated with a high risk of complications," he said.

"For this reason there is general agreement that new types of ablation systems designed specifically to create continuous linear lesions are needed."

Private enterprise once more into the breach, so began the process of catapulting a new generation of medical technology into to the market place–ready or not.

Funding flowed from Silicon Valley and Wall Street into start-up businesses, and established medical device companies spun off new divisions. Qualified R&D professionals were in high demand. Members of the EP research community rented themselves out to device manufactures. Goats and pigs and dogs were catheterized and cauterized, and the study data was analyzed. Techniques and theories were tried and abandoned as new ablation systems proliferated.

Collectively, the journal articles from the period convey a sense of anticipation, an anxious groping for the cure, and excitement at the prospect of being first in the field.

Chapter 6

The Cat's out of the Bag

THE UNITED STATES Food and Drug Administration, watching the parade of medical progress from the sidelines, looked for a way to assert its authority. Great strides were being made in America's electrophysiology labs, and regulators needed to catch up. The overburdened staff at the FDA was always at least a step behind medical advances in the field, which seemed to come faster everyday. Both the pace of technology and the wily ways of device manufacturers kept it that way.

Boston Scientific, a global corporation with more than 13,000 devices in its product line, knows the regulatory ropes. According to a Hoover's profile, "Boston Scientific would typically introduce a device for use in less critical places, such as the urinary tract, and then apply it to higher-risk situations, such as those in cardiology. This helped speed up development of new products."

The speedy development of new products led to the inevitable use of those new products, often in imaginative and unproven ways; using a device "off label" is the legal and accepted way to expand its scope and revenue potential. Despite the lack of FDA approval, cardiac catheter ablation devices were being widely and routinely deployed in patients across the country in attempts to treat specific conditions, and the new quest for the Afib cure was about to greatly expand that practice.

Something had to be done. Regulators decided to raise the bar for approval of catheter ablation devices used in treating atrial fibrillation, and the less complicated condition of atrial flutter.

Up until now, new devices could be approved with a 510k letter from the FDA, which meant that if you could demonstrate that your ablation catheter was pretty much the same as the one already on the market, you could skip the tough questions about safety and efficacy.

The agency stamped your device as being "substantially equivalent" to the previous model, and then you were free to set the sales force loose on physicians and patients.

Now that the FDA was requiring that devices to treat specific arrhythmias be proven safe and effective through use in clinical trials, it had to figure out exactly how those clinical trials should be designed.

So, in the long, hot summer days toward the end of July 1998, the FDA's Circulatory System Devices Panel summoned researchers, device makers, and doctors to the Gaithersburg Holiday Inn near Rockville, Maryland to help craft new rules for the new century of medicine. Such a big crowd was expected that they opened up the Grand Ballroom, which is what you get when you fold up the wall that divides the Goshen Room from the Potomac Room.

To kick off the first of a series of meetings, the panel's Executive Secretary, FDA cardiologist John Stuhlmuller, gave the mandatory reading of the conflict of interest statement. He noted that sometimes a member's value to the panel outweighed any perceived conflicts, and these people get waivers.

Practically everyone who worked in Rockville had been granted a conflict of interest waiver at one time or another. To be fair, they have to do that as a practical matter. Most cardiologists who consult for the FDA get speaking fees, grants, consultation fees and medical advisory fees from all the big companies.

If candidates were excluded from regulatory panels based upon their financial arrangements with medical device manufacturers, you'd never get a quorum.

Not to say there is anything unseemly going on.

Dr. Cynthia Tracy runs the cardiology shop at George Washington University.

A veteran stalker of the these halls, she knew the names of all the meeting rooms of the Gaithersburg Holiday Inn and had learned, from long, tedious stretches in each and everyone one of them and their various permutations to get right to the point.

But now she was having trouble conveying her thoughts on the matter at hand.

And who could blame her?

The FDA determines a device's classification by its intended use and the risk that the device presents to the patient.

New medical devices are compared to legally marketed medical devices with the same intended use.

The regulatory hall of mirrors in which the panel members found themselves was illustrated by the situation with catheter ablation for atrial flutter, which was being routinely performed with off-label devices.

All new catheters coming on the market to treat a-flutter would henceforth have to be approved specifically for that purpose.

Approval meant making sure they were at least as good as what was already out there.

What was already out there were catheters not approved for a-flutter and were therefore being used off-label, which meant that they were investigational devices—and you cannot approve an investigational device by comparing it to another investigational device.

Tracy didn't see any way out. "It's all done off-label," she noted, "but the reality is that we are doing this procedure everyday. Everybody is. People are using off-label catheters very successfully to perform catheter ablation of atrial flutter. I don't see how we can ignore the fact."

Someone floated the idea of doing a clinical study using existing catheter systems and established practices; a study to evaluate and approve an already proven procedure, thereby sanctifying the status quo. It would be sort of like Congress authorizing the sun to come up yesterday.

Tracy couldn't begin to conceive of a rationalization for it.

"I don't think that is going to fly in any sense, because the cat is out of the bag with that," she said, "and clinical practice is clinical practice at this point. I think we are too far down the road to turn our backs to that fact," Tracy said.

Chapter 7

Not so Fast

> *3/25/02 14:08 Nursing Note: "Patient more alert. Patient is at present unwilling to proceed to surgery. Cardiac surgery, CCU attending in to discuss with pt and family."*

PAM'S MAIDEN NAME, as they used to say, is Johnson, and as she lay there in the CCU anesthetized and oblivious to the impending bad news, I kept thinking of this joke:

An Army sergeant calls a PFC in to tell him that he's just been promoted to squad leader, and his first assignment is to tell Private Johnson that his mother died. The new squad leader assembles the company and says "Everyone whose mother is still alive, take one step forward... NOT SO FAST THERE, JOHNSON!"

And at first Pam thought I was joking, the sort of gallows humor that gets people through hospital visits. Here she was expecting to be going home, having gone through a bit of an ordeal, but at least she'd gotten it over with. Her Afib would be cured. "Listen," I said. "There really was a problem... " The idea didn't sink in slowly, it just struck, and when it did, something in her crumpled and her head sank back into the pillow, stunned, staring at the ceiling, her eyes welling up.

After a time, she turned angry and her expression turned to one of grim determination: She would not consent to open-heart surgery. This is a woman who has seen many an oozing chest wound.

"They screwed up a pacemaker, a catheterization and now I'm supposed to let them cut me, open me up? Open-heart surgery? No. No. No. I won't do it."

The bed sheets were knotted in clenched fists over her chest as if for protection against the thought.

And I had to admit she had me there. Except for the looming death sentence implicit in her refusal, her position made perfect sense.

A little later we joked about calling an ambulance to get her out of Hopkins and take her over to George Washington Hospital—and boy do I wish now that we had really done that.

To be fair to Johns Hopkins, it was Dr. Grant Simons in Annapolis who screwed up the pacemaker job. He poked a hole—actually in the business they call it a *microperforation*—in Pam's heart with a pacemaker lead, *microperf* for short. Having worked in politics, I was up on all the government type euphemisms; friendly fire, underprivileged, etc., but I was learning the medical lexicon now. *Microperf.* One would think that the wall of a human heart would have to be either perfed or not perfed.

Both the *microperf* and what happened to Pam in the Hopkins EP lab were *complications*. And, since there was a war on, and military euphemisms were in the air, Professor Calkins would later borrow a phrase to describe Pam's contribution to the advancement of medical science. He would refer to my wife Pam as *collateral damage*. I discovered much later that the *microperfing* of Pam's heart in 1998 was the *complication* that led to her becoming part of *the learning curve* and ultimately to be classified as *collateral damage* in 2002.

Speaking of euphemisms, I find that it does not pay to write that someone lied. People don't like the word.

So I use a word that lawyers use to describe someone who is lying, obfuscating or otherwise not telling the truth. They say the respondent is dancing. You wouldn't think it to look at him, but I found out that the head of the EP Lab at Johns Hopkins Medicine can dance like Fred Astaire.

In any event, Pam was serious about not consenting to open-heart surgery. She just wasn't going to do it.

Although I never once thought about just letting her die, I did have to acknowledge her right to refuse, and to recognize her feelings as legitimate.

Because of her experiences in nursing and the drawn out hospital deaths of both of our fathers, we had discussed the rights of people to just say no. No more torture just let me go.

She had that right and I had to respect that. But she also had a son and a daughter and the rest of her family and me–and whatever lay ahead she was just going to have to go through it.

She closed her eyes. I let her hand go and went out into the hall to tell the surgeon that she will do it, just give me some time.

He looked me in the eye.

"We're out of time."

Around the same time that the FDA's Circulatory Systems Devices Approval Panel was booking rooms in Gaithersburg for the big series of meetings in 1998, Pam went to see a cardiologist in Annapolis because of occasional fainting and dizziness. It was determined from a series of tests that she had a condition called Syncope and that a pacemaker was in order.

Annapolis electrophysiologist Grant Simons would implant it. We met with Dr. Simons. He is a pleasant man with an easy smile. We both liked him, and Pam took his advice.

"Successful implantation of a dual chamber pacemaker," he exclaimed in his report of the procedure that summer, and that's definitely where he wanted to leave it.

Pam would have preferred that version of reality as well, but there was a problem.

She was doing fine in the hospital when I went to pick her up, all smiles and I'm glad that's over with. I was going to take her to our favorite little neighborhood restaurant. She signed the forms, changed into her street clothes, declined the wheel chair, and said thanks and good night to all. And then she walked out into the hallway and collapsed. Nurses and aides rushed over.

We formed a circle around her there on the floor. I remember someone slapping her hand, saying "Come on honey, wake up..." And Pam did wake up and she said, "I almost passed out."

The nurse said "you did pass out, honey," and there on the floor, Pam began to cry. She raised her right hand to her left shoulder, which was covered by a sling. "I thought this was all over," she said.

A nurse got hold of the cardiologist on call, who had them check out the pacemaker. Upon hearing that it was working fine, the doctor said that it was OK with him if Pam went home. So I took her home. The first thing she did was run to the nearest bathroom in the house and start retching and heaving.

I called the cardiology group. A few minutes later, the covering doc was on the phone. He sounded like he'd been interrupted. He sounded annoyed. I said I just got Pam home from the hospital and she is violently ill. He said that wasn't possible.

He said that the only way Pam could be that sick would be if a pacemaker lead had perforated her heart and no such thing had occurred here. Pam was probably ill from the anesthesia, get a prescription filled and she'll be OK.

She rode out the night on swells of nausea.

Then she began to get a feeling like she was being poked in the ribs by a hot needle with every beat of her heart—which was pretty much what was happening.

The tips of pacemaker leads are designed to screw into the wall of the heart. If they get screwed in too far, they go through the heart and send little jolts to the chest wall muscles.

But if the chest wall muscles were being paced, that would mean that Grant Simons had poked a hole in Pam's heart. And that just can't be. So Simons elected to adjust the pacemaker settings and change her medications in the hope that he could somehow make the problem go away.

In choosing to deal with the error by adjusting settings along with the doses and types of medication, Simons had set Pam on the path to Room One at the Hopkins EP Lab.

The procedure was performed on a 50-year old man and the family was initially told by the surgeon that the surgery went well. While recovering in his room the patient went into cardiac arrest and a code blue was called. Despite resuscitative efforts the patient was unable to breathe for about twenty minutes and a CT scan showed that because of the prolonged deprivation of oxygen the patient suffered profound irreversible brain injury.

Chapter 8
Just because you can doesn't mean you should

"As we sit comfortably in the dawn of the 21st century, reflecting on how much we know today compared with our investigative grandfathers in the early and mid portions of the 20th century, we should surely not get too complacent or too smug; for certain, our investigative great grandchildren 50 to 100 years from now will be surprised at how little we knew regarding the mechanism of atrial fibrillation and approaches to its treatment."

– Eric N. Prystowsky, M.D.

A HUNDRED YEARS from now? The cardiologists meeting at the Holiday Inn back in 1998 to assess the state of the electrophysiological arts weren't surprised at how little they knew; they *knew* how little they knew.

When the device approval panel discussed the merits of catheter ablation for atrial fibrillation, Dr. J. Marcus Wharton, M.D., as he is redundantly tagged on the website of the Medical University of South Carolina, began by pointing out that there was a gaping hole in the basic theory.

You had to do more than merely relieve symptoms with an invasive and risky procedure like catheter ablation, Wharton said, because "we can relieve the symptoms with drugs."

"And the thing is," he added, "if we eliminate symptoms and appear to have fixed the underlying condition, an assumption is going to be made by the practicing physician that they can stop warfarin on that patient," which would be setting the patient up for a stroke if and when the Afib silently resumed.

Just because you couldn't feel it anymore didn't mean that you could stop taking your blood thinning medication. A lack of symptoms didn't mean your heart chambers were now all working in perfect synchronization, keeping the blood flowing smoothly enough to prevent a clot from forming that could kill you–or worse.

Medically speaking, the term *morbidity* relates to people getting sick from a particular treatment or drug, and there is a lot of morbidity associated with taking warfarin. "So the bigger issue is," said Wharton, "can I do something that would allow me to take someone off of warfarin." If people could stop taking the harsh drug, which prevented a stroke–a *cerebral vascular accident* in the lexicon of the lab– an ablation might be worth the risks. On the other hand, the main risk of an ablation procedure is having a stroke.

"So I think that we are going to have to look very closely at what we are doing," Wharton said.

"I couldn't agree more," said Dr. Tracy. "We really have to understand why we are doing this in the first place. Right now, this is such an unknown thing to me. I am a real skeptic. I don't know why we are talking about this whole thing in the first place, anyway," she said.

Tracy couldn't get over it. "We would have to go a long way before I would be convinced that we are achieving better than what we can do with warfarin therapy. So why are we doing this in the first place? I don't know. But I sure know that I don't want this to be done and to have anybody made worse," she said.

She knew, though, why they were all there, and she had concerns about it. "We're really pushing the technology," she said. "Just because you can, doesn't mean you should. We are struggling to figure out exactly what it is that needs to be done. We don't even know.

"We don't know anything about what lesions we really need, anything about what locations you need. We don't know anything about it at all, as far as I am concerned. So I think it makes designing a study very, very difficult because we don't know very much about even what it is that we are trying to accomplish.

"We don't know anything. I don't know why we are talking about this whole thing in the first place."

This got Dr. Anne Curtis, the Panel Chair, to thinking about lesion sets, what configuration of scars might work best against Afib, and where exactly in the heart they should be placed. "You're right," Curtis said. "I don't believe anyone has quite worked out what the lesion sets are. I would have to say I don't know. Nobody knows."

The EP community tried hard to solve that puzzle over the next few years, branding many configurations into many hearts. These included:

Linear ablation at the mitral isthmus.

Linear block at the left atrial roof.

Left atrial junction disconnect.

Cavotricuspid isthmus ablation.

Catheter ablation of cardiac autonomic nerves.

Focal pulmonary vein isolation.

Segmental pulmonary vein isolation.

Circumferential pulmonary vein isolation.

Linear ablation of the isthmus between the inferior vena cava and tricuspid annulus.

Then there was the famous Kitchen Sink Combo: A randomized study comparing combined pulmonary vein-left atrial junction disconnection and cavotricuspid isthmus ablation versus pulmonary vein-left atrial junction disconnection alone.

And it all started in the right atrium. Whether or not it should have was a controversial question, which Panel Chair Anne Curtis dutifully posed to those assembled in the Grand Ballroom. They were moving right along that afternoon.

"Question Number 14," she read, "Is it appropriate to begin an Afib study in the right heart only, in order to characterize the safety of the device in a lower-risk environment or can patients be treated in the left heart with a new ablation system without any right heart experience?"

Curtis put in that she wasn't comfortable with the implications of the question as stated, and Dr. Simmons agreed. "It implies you are doing a lesser procedure just to find out what the risks are," he said.

"That's right," said Dr. Curtis.

But Dr. Wharton saw an advantage to the right-side only approach. "There is a huge learning curve with the investigator with any new catheter and I think, in terms of safety," he said, "that it is probably better for them to learn in the right atrium where there is less they can hurt, before we start sticking... "

That's as far as Wharton got before Anne Curtis cut in, pointing out that "that means you are using the patient to get your learning curve in."

As that concept was settling over the medicine men in the Grand Ballroom, the voice of conscience arose from an unlikely corner.

"My name is Michael Ross," said a young man in the back of the room. "I am from industry, a company called Atrionics, working specifically in catheter ablation of atrial arrhythmias. I remain a little confused on this right-sided, left-sided, debate. Because if you look at the results of right-sided ablating over the past couple of years, I think that, at best, the companies that have released their results are operating at the margins and, at worst, I would say that the data from these studies would probably never pass FDA scrutiny." When it came to atrial fibrillation, right-sided ablation was practically useless.

Mike Ross had their attention and he pressed ahead.

"We are moving from the question, will right-sided lesions work, to are they needed at all... but the more important fact is that left-sided lesions are almost certainly needed," Ross said.

"So it begs the question. How do you consent a patient for a right-sided-only procedure and is it ethical to do? How do we go to these patients and tell them we are going to do a procedure on the right side, that it is probably not going to work, but we just need to get this data?"

I'll tell you how, said Dr. George Vetrovec, the Chairman of the Cardiology Department at Virginia Commonwealth University and part owner of four medical companies. "There have been a number of trials in all kinds of things where the first three procedures done in each investigator's institution are done a specific way. In this case, it would be right-sided-only ablations," Vetrovec said, explaining that once investigators had duly demonstrated that right sided ablation was ineffective (with acceptable casualty rates), it would then be technically ethical to start in on the left side.

"But," objected Dr. Tracy, "We know it is potentially a very unsafe procedure. If the success is not likely to be very high with right-sided lesions only, then it doesn't make sense to limit a study to right-sided lesions only."

"Can't argue with that," said Dr. Wharton.

"Well," said Dr. Salim Aziz, a cardiac surgeon from Denver, "You will have a learning curve of doctors learning to use the catheter, and this is a point where you are gathering data, so if the patients are willing to take that chance..."

Dr. Tony Simmons, speaking for the United States Food and Drug Administration, nipped that whole idea right in the bud. "To submit a patient to a right-sided ablation just to get practice is not going to happen," he said, "It is not going to happen."

Actually, it already was happening.

––––––––––

Hugh Calkins, working for Guidant Inc., published an article in The American Journal of Cardiology in the spring of 1999 about what he did last summer–while the gang in Gaithersburg was busy making up the rules:

A New System for Catheter Ablation of Atrial Fibrillation

> A prospective multicenter clinical trial to evaluate the safety and efficacy of a right atrial ablation procedure to treat atrial fibrillation is currently underway using the Guidant Heart Rhythm Technologies Linear Ablation System. To date, 15 patients have been enrolled, and the procedure was acutely effective in 14 of 15 patients with no complications.

> Atrial fibrillation has recurred during short-term follow-up in 12 of 15 patients, a not surprising result, because this initial phase of testing involved only right-sided ablation. The early results of the phase I clinical trial confirm the findings of others that successful ablation of chronic atrial fibrillation is likely to require a left atrial approach."

And they said it couldn't be done. Well, actually they said submitting a patient to a risky right-sided ablation procedure just to gather data and get some practice shouldn't be done, that it would never be done.

But you can't stop progress.

The catch phrase for medical device regulation had just been altered to "safe *or* effective," and eventually, after a bidding war with Johnson & Johnson, the Guidant Corporation was bought by Boston Scientific, Inc. for $27 billion in cash.

the doctor put the catheder up through my groin and into my left (i think) heart valve. When he put the catheder in through the valve the catheder became tangled on one of the chordae that helps hold the valve shut. The doctor tried to get the catheder untangled and ended up damaging/tearing one of the chordae on that valve.

The doctor told my parents that they were sending the catheder out to "engineering" to find out if there was something wrong with it because they have never had this happen before in all of the heart ablations that they have done. The doctor said it was probably just because my anatomy was different and he really couldnt explain why this happened.

I dont have health insurance because im 24 and never thought that i would have heart problems at this age and i was going to pay for this ablation myself with my own money. Well now that this is happened i will have to pay for the ablation that they didnt do because they had to stop and ill have to pay for being in the hospital for longer. Then, ill have to go back and get the ablation done a 2nd time AND get my heart valve fixed.

Chapter 9

The Bottom Line

JOHNS HOPKINS fosters a cozy relationship with the corporate world, and device manufacturers cozied right up when catheter ablation for atrial fibrillation looked to be the next hot investment. Professor Calkins, the pioneer in right-sided ablations for Afib, had been collaborating with companies like Johnson & Johnson, Medtronic and St. Jude Medical on various techniques and technologies since the mid 1990's. He'd also done business with Biosense Webster, Ablation Frontiers, Boston Scientific, ProRhythm, IRhythm, CryoCor, Reliant, Bard, Guidant, Sanofi Aventis, CyberHeart and a company called AtriCure.

Of these companies, Medtronic, Boston Scientific, Guidant, Atricure and St. Jude caught the attention of the U.S. Justice Department for paying kickbacks to doctors to use their ablation devices, bilking millions from Medicare in the process.

And, in a strange twist, Calkins sits on "The Medical Advisory Board" for TASER International. TASER's only product, a stun gun, has been known to actually cause fatal arrhythmias.

Hugh Calkins is paid to say it ain't necessarily so. It's like the teacher who was being considered for a job, and the school board wanted to know whether he would teach that the world was round or flat.

He said he could teach it either way.

Just when the cash started to really roll in for TASER shareholders and executives, a 14-year-old boy took a jolt from a cop in Chicago and died. *CBS News* did an investigative story on TASER, casting doubt on the integrity of safety studies designed to help sell law enforcement on the weapon.

With deaths steadily mounting and, worse, becoming increasingly publicized, the company needed some big names to vouch for the safety of the TASER, so they went out and bought them, along with the prestige of Johns Hopkins Medicine. In addition to Hugh Calkins, they recruited high-profile cardiologist Richard Luceri from the University of Miami. Luceri and Calkins became the TASER twins of American cardiology.

Their safety studies showed up in medical journals–for later distribution as TASER propaganda.

Press conferences were called and interviews were arranged. An authoritative Hugh Grosvenor Calkins, MD–Johns Hopkins Medicine writ large on his lab coat–was trotted out to reporters around the country with the message that TASER studies were sound as a dollar. He pronounced the device to be perfectly safe, supplying reams of incomprehensible data on troponin levels and biomarkers and baseline studies—to television reporters.

The endorsement was used as a legal defense in a securities fraud lawsuit filed in Arizona in which company execs were charged with dumping stock before passing news of legal troubles on to stockholders:

Dr. Hugh Calkins, Professor of Medicine and Director of the Arrhythmia Service at Johns Hopkins Hospital, concluded, "I have had an opportunity to review the studies and the results of the studies confirm the general safety of the TASER devices, and I personally believe this technology is saving lives everyday."

Since that pronouncement, Amnesty International says that more than 330 people have died after TASER attacks in the US and Canada.

The debate in the medical journals took some interesting turns. Dr. Zian Tseng, a cardiologist and electrophysiologist at UCSF who specializes in heart-rhythm disorders, told reporter Alan Gathright of the *San Francisco Chronicle* "I've seen the TASER folks say, 'Oh, the guy had cocaine in his system, that's the reason for his death.' Well, someone with cocaine in their system is also much more prone to a TASER-induced cardiac arrest. They cannot say that it's safe in my opinion."

Au contraire, replied Hugh Calkins, asserting that a generous helping of nose candy would actually make for a safer–if not more thrilling–TASER experience.

"It is erroneous to state that the presence of cocaine makes an electronic control device more dangerous.," Calkins said. "Cocaine is a strong sodium-channel blocker... the net effect is to increase the threshold for ventricular fibrillation, not lower it."

A study in the American Journal of Cardiology undercut TASER's claim that stun guns made it less dangerous for police to arrest violent suspects–without risk to alleged perpetrators. "Although considered by some a safer alternative to firearms, TASER deployment was associated with a substantial increase in in-custody sudden deaths, with no decrease officer injuries." Just the opposite of the bought and paid for professional opinion TASER Inc. was waiving around in the media and using to legally challenge candid medical examiners.

TASER, Inc. has waged a vigorous campaign to make sure that the phrases "electronic control device" and "cause of death" never meet in public. Robert Anglen at the *Arizona Republic* reported on how vigorously the company challenged physicians who blamed the TASER for a death:

> A Chicago medical examiner has ruled that shocks from a TASER were responsible for the death of a man in February, marking the first time that the electronic stun gun has been named as the primary cause of death.
>
> This is the latest challenge to Scottsdale-based TASER International's claim that its stun guns have never caused a death or serious injury and comes a week after an Illinois police department filed a class-action lawsuit claiming TASER misled law enforcement agencies about the safety of its weapon.
>
> The death is the 18th case in which a coroner has cited TASER as a factor in someone's death and the fourth case where TASER has been named as a cause of death.
>
> But in all of those, TASER was secondary to other factors such as drugs, heart conditions or mental illness.
>
> TASER strongly criticized the Medical Examiner's Office in a statement Friday and said it will challenge the autopsy. "We believe that the scientific and medical community will publicly challenge this conclusion based upon the lack of credible evidence," TASER spokesman Steve Tuttle wrote in an e-mail on Friday. "TASER International will seek a judicial review of the report and the basis for which those statements were made."
>
> This is not the first time TASER has challenged a medical examiner. For years, TASER officials publicly said the stun gun was never cited in an autopsy report. But an Arizona Republic investigation last year

revealed that TASERs have been cited repeatedly by medical examiners in death cases and that TASER did not start collecting autopsy reports until last April.

When Dr. Lisa Kohler, chief medical examiner in Summit County, Ohio, listed stun gun use as a contributing factor in three deaths, TASER sued, forcing Kohler to delete any such reference from her reports. The National Association of Medical Examiners protested, calling the move "dangerously close to intimidation."

Then came the death by TASER of a disoriented Polish immigrant named Robert Dziekański at the hands of police at Vancouver International Airport, which was caught on video.

The story immediately attained the satellite news orbit and began playing out 24 hours a day all around the world. Calkins and Luceri stuck by their assertion that such deaths were caused by a conjured-up malady called "Excited Delirium," which has been ridiculed as a mythical condition and a dubious disorder by those not on the TASER pad.

That was enough for Canadians. Canadian doctors, anyway. An editorial in the Journal of the Canadian Medical Association heaped scorn on scientists and physicians who got paid to defend the company:

> "TASER International appears to attract loyalty. The scientific literature bears witness to a small group of dedicated researchers who diligently write letters to journals pointing out flaws in studies reporting harm from TASERs. Unfortunately, some of these researchers occasionally neglect to mention their participation on TASER International's medical advisory board or board of directors…"

The editorial ended with the statement that "We are used to thinking like physicians and scientists concerned about health, preferring to gather and analyze the facts rather than succumbing to the bald assertions of a large corporate entity that has demonstrated a willingness to squelch any messages that could hurt its bottom line."

Chapter 10
The Alive or Dead Thing

THE LASSO CATHETER that Richard Wu corkscrewed into the left ventricle of Pam's heart was a mapping device, designed to figure out where the burns from the ablation catheter should be applied. The Lasso mapping catheter was manufactured by Johnson & Johnson Inc., which keeps Hugh Calkins more or less on retainer and pays the salaries of the cardiology fellows at Hopkins.

To make the scars inside Pam's heart, Wu was "learning by burning" with the Chilli Cooled-tip ablation catheter. One big problem with cardiac catheter ablations, which they discovered as the procedures got more and more popular, was that blood tended to coagulate near the hot tip of the catheter, resulting in clots and strokes. The Chilli, a water-cooled catheter developed by Cardiac Pathways, was designed to overcome the problem.

Cardiac Pathways was an emerging medical device company with a lot of potential and not much else. The company sought approval for its new product at one of the FDA meetings held in the Grand Ballroom in the summer of 1998.

Here's what went into the company prospectus:

> "Since inception, the Company has been primarily engaged in researching, developing, testing—and obtaining regulatory clearances for—mapping and ablation catheters, equipment and systems. These catheter and equipment systems are currently the Company's only significant potential products."

Here was the strategy the company laid out to produce and sell actual products:

> "The Company intends to build on relationships with electrophysiologists. The Company has developed strong relationships with prominent electrophysiologists worldwide who have been involved and will continue to be involved in the Company's clinical and product development.
>
> The Company intends to continue to build these substantial relationships through clinical investigator meetings, participation in physician-run symposia and meetings to discuss clinical issues and treatments. The Company's strategy is to leverage these relationships with leading electrophysiologists to gain market acceptance of its products in the United States and internationally."

It was a cultivated, compensated, and presumably leveraged Hugh Calkins who represented Cardiac Pathways before the FDA in its bid to get the Chilli cooled-tip catheter approved. Dr. Jeff Brinker, a Calkins underling at Hopkins, was a voting member of the FDA panel that day. He had been granted a waiver.

The Chilli cooled-tip catheter was approved—despite questions about the statistical vagaries of the clinical trial and the staggering body count left in its wake.

The question before Jeff Brinker and the rest of the FDA panel that day was whether or not a Chilli cooled-tip ablation procedure was safe and effective. Cardiac Pathways proposed labeling cooled-tip ablation as a low-risk procedure, which didn't sit well with panel member Dr. Cynthia Tracy.

"I think that's something that we are going to have to reconsider," she said, "given that complications occurred in 44 out of 150 patients."

The death toll at the end of the study, depending on your statistical dexterity, amounted to more than two dozen people, and at least six of those patients died as a direct result of undergoing the procedure.

Calkins reported that the first patient cut down by the learning curve was a 63-year-old man. Thirty minutes after they started burning, a blood clot plugged the left main coronary artery of his heart. His blood pressure bottomed out and he died of cardiogenic shock. The second casualty came when a catheter was poked through the heart wall of a 72-year-old man. His blood pressure collapsed also, and he died a week later. Next, a 74-year-old man was killed when a catheter wire ripped his aortic valve apart.

Then a 49-year-old man "underwent a successful ablation, but suffered a cerebrovascular accident that progressed to herniation and death," according to Calkins. In other words, during the procedure, a blood vessel had burst in this 49-year-old man's brain, and the pressure in his skull built up so much that it pushed his brain stem down into his spinal column. The patient died, but the ablation went on the books as a success.

FDA Panel member Dr. Tony Simmons of Wake Forest University recommended that Cardiac Pathways change the patient counseling information for the Chilli cooled-tip ablation catheter "to more accurately reflect the risk and the lack of demonstrated effectiveness overall."

Dr. Simmons, who had determined that the Chilli catheter was no improvement over similar products already on the market, was curious about the reasons for the study's high casualty rate. "I would have thought that, well, when a significant percentage of the patients died, I mean... there should have been some autopsy data, right?"

Maybe there should have been, but there wasn't.

Even though it was his Hopkins boss Hugh Calkins asking him to approve the Chilli catheter, panel member Jeff Brinker had trouble squaring the lack of safety data.

They didn't really get any insights from the clinical trial, and you really couldn't trust the professional journal articles to assess the risks, Brinker said, because in the literature, "people sort of cherry pick what they do, and they write that up."

To really find out how risky this thing was, you'd have to "get a bigger denominator," he said. "So, I think that we just need a couple of hundred patients who get an ablation so we can really look at what the procedural risk is."

Brinker wanted Cardiac Pathways, once the procedure was established practice, to conduct post-market surveillance, which meant keeping a running casualty list and periodically reporting it to the FDA. You'd find out how risky it was once doctors across the country started doing the procedure by the hundreds. Just get it out there and let them start doing it and see what happens.

"Do you mean," asked Dr. Simmons, "a follow-up on the alive or dead thing?"

Just so, said Brinker.

And that's what they did. With little evidence of its safety or effectiveness, and despite the lack of autopsy data on those who died so that others could make a killing, the Chilli cooled-tip catheter was approved, and it went on to enjoy great financial success in the marketplace as a device to treat atrial fibrillation (off-label).

Boston Scientific, Inc. eventually bought Cardiac Pathways for $115 million in cash.

Is there anyone out there that has hypertrophic cardiomyopathy and was told to have an ablation? Any problems??? My husband of 45years and I believed that his cardio doctor would not put him in harms way by letting an associate/dr. perform this procedure which was nothing short of a disaster.

After he came out of surgery dr. said he would be in recovery room for two hours and go home..... We couldn't even get him up in two hours.....I asked the nurse to get him some jello so I could get something in his stomach when we got him up....

When she helped get him up and I fed him a few spoonfulls he laid his head back on the pillow a few seconds later blood was coming out the sides of his mouth..... The 5 family members ran in the hall to get the nurse, she started phoning doctor,,, He answered page after two hours then told her he would be down in a few minutes ...

She came back in the room 45 minutes later and sadly told us Dr....... went HOME..... anyhow things got worst....The two hour procedure plus two hour recovery room wound up being six days the doctor never stepped foot in my husbands room all the days he was in that hospital. The day he left that doctors assistant brought in an appointment for 3 months later.... My husband was never the same again....He passed away 5 weeks later..

The Cardiac Pathways acquisition would prove to be a much better move for Boston Scientific than its subsequent $27 billion cash purchase of Guidant Corporation, which turned out to be one of the biggest big money fiascoes of the decade. Guidant's Heart Rhythm Technologies Linear Ablation System, which Hugh Calkins had unveiled as the big advance over the drag and burn technique, mysteriously fizzled, its secrets buried deep in government files under many layers of Freedom of Information Act requests. It was totally forgotten in the waves of corruption scandals and the high-volume product failures that came with the Guidant purchase, scandals which would shake the very foundations of the Boston Scientific empire.

Calkins, however, had his linear ablation bases covered. Even as the plug was being pulled on Guidant's Heart Rhythm system, he was working with rival company Cardima (Cardiac Rhythm Disorder Management) Inc., to help develop the REVELATION linear catheter ablation system, which was similar in design and purpose.

Cardima was a Silicon Valley start up with high hopes and $3 million from investors. Their REVELATION system was supposed to be the new defining step up from the drag and burn. Its main attraction, as with the Guidant system, was an ablation catheter with electrodes lined up one behind another along the end so you could just lay it against the heart wall and burn the entire single line at once. For whatever—or whomever—it was worth, you could supposedly make straight, neat, continuous lines of scar tissue in the right atrium with the REVELATION catheter ablation system.

Cardima's stock price nearly doubled in 1998 on the announcement that the REVELATION system had been approved in Europe. The company immediately began laying the groundwork for approval in the U.S., beginning with dog studies. Hugh Calkins started giving Baltimore's Chinatown competition for the city's mongrel population.

Many a stray has been sacrificed on the altar of science at Hopkins, the canines in this case delivered up in order to fulfill the requisite animal study phase on the road to clinical trials on humans.

The results of the canine study were duly published in one of the EP trade journals and Calkins reported that Cardima's REVELATION catheter system performed magnificently. (On the Internet, Cardima files their copy of the article under Assets/Calkins.) The company parlayed the successful results of the dog study into FDA approval for a clinical trial using human beings. There was politics; the company successfully lobbied the FDA to expedite the review process—on pretty shaky ground. Despite Hugh Calkins's famous acknowledgment that "nobody ever died from Afib," the FDA granted the company's request on the grounds that the device treated a condition that was "life threatening" and there was no other option available to patients.

As soon as the investigational studies were approved and underway, the REVELATION system was promoted at cardiology meetings and in magazine articles and ads. Business press releases heralded advances along the way, breathing life into the company stock and soothing anxious investors.

Chapter 11

And Yes I said Yes I Will Yes

> "A perfunctory signing of a consent form elicits mere passive assent, not active consent. It neither enhances patient understanding nor helps the patient take responsibility for his or her choices. There is a substantial consensus in our society that it is unethical to impose risks on people without their consent."
>
> *– Dr. Harold J. Bursztajn*

YES.

What else could you say?

Here, with the blanks filled in, is the form I gave Pam to sign when she finally consented to open-heart surgery:

I hereby give my consent and authorize Doctor *Yuh/Cameron* of the Johns Hopkins Hospital to perform the following operation or other procedure: *Mitral Valve Repair/Mitral Valve Replacement Possible Removal of Right Ventricular pacing lead*

The nature and purpose of the operation or other procedure and anesthesia, the risks involved have been explained. *Doctor Walinsky* has explained alternatives and the possibility of complications to me. **I am aware that the practice of medicine and surgery is not an exact science and I acknowledge that no guarantee has been made as to the results that may be obtained.** (Emphasis added.) All my questions, if any, have been answered to my satisfaction.

If Pam wasn't aware that the practice of medicine and surgery at Johns Hopkins was not an exact science when we drove up to the place that morning, she sure became aware of it over the course of the next three and a half weeks.

Here is the informed consent supplement:

1. Indications for the operation: *Acutely Leaking Heart Valve*
2. Risks: *Bleeding, Infection, Heart Attack, Stroke, Death*
3. Alternatives to the Proposed Operation: *Not to Operate*

Well, there you have it, sign and maybe die, or don't sign and definitely die. It's your choice, and either way you can't blame Johns Hopkins. I was holding a clipboard and a pen out to my wife as she stared at the ceiling.

Her eyelashes were wet. She blinked, and a tear rolled from the corner of her eye straight down the side of her face into the pillow.

"A discussion of the risks, benefits, and alternatives should be undertaken in an unpressured environment well before the procedure... It is better to explain the potential risks, benefits, and alternative therapies to coronary intervention before administration of sedatives or other agents that may affect the patient's judgment."

So sayeth the American College of Cardiology about informed consent.

I'm no expert, but it seems to me that gathering a signature from someone who's doped up and crying because she's literally just had part of her heart ripped out and who has been told to sign or die, well it seems to me that violates the spirit of the ACC directive on informed consent. But what do I know?

The main thing for these guys was to get the name on the dotted line.

I didn't discuss the possibility of mitral valve replacement with Pam. When she took the pen from my hand to make the understandably half-hearted scrawl near the signature line before she was lifted up out of the bed and on to the gurney.

I am here to tell you that she did not care much for fine print.

She had not read any of it, and so would not have seen the part about mitral valve replacement instead of repair.

Repairing a valve as opposed to replacing it with a prosthetic valve makes a big difference in your life, and I knew it. But I didn't say anything to her about that—nor did any of the surgeons.

(Pam still finds it remarkable that Hugh Calkins left her on the surgeon's doorstep and skulked away, leaving it to others to explain her new medical status.)

Drs. Walinsky, Yuh and Cameron are all honorable men and skilled physicians as far as I knew—and as far as I still know. But under the circumstances, I couldn't recall if any of them were the surgeons we'd met, and neither Pam nor I knew anything of their skills or their backgrounds and experience.

But they had a signed consent form and she had no choice, so off she went. I squeezed her hand and gave her a kiss as she was wheeled down the hall flat on her back and then was gone behind the big, black double doors, away to the Operating Room— wherever that was.

> *"The patient's chest, abdomen and lower extremities were prepped and draped... After a median sternotomy incision was made, the sternum was divided with a bone saw... Reasonable exposure of the mitral valve apparatus was noted. The valve leaflets were intact; however, the posterior leaflet was completely flail due to separation of the posteromedial papillary muscle near its base.*

> *"Moreover, two chordae on the remnant tip of the papillary muscle were also severed. It appeared unlikely that an adequate repair could be accomplished in this setting. Therefore, the anterior leaflet was excised along its chordal attachments, and the medial scallop of the posterior leaflet was also excised..."*

> — Yuh, David

Accepting the fact that Pam signed a standard consent form in the stressful moments before the ablation procedure, the form contains no such language as is offered at other hospitals:

> I authorize Dr. _____, and such physicians in training and assistants as (s)he may select, to treat my condition... **I UNDERSTAND THAT PHYSICIANS IN TRAINING MAY PERFORM PORTIONS OF THE PROCEDURES DESCRIBED BELOW** ..." [Emphasis Original] University of Virginia Health System.

Contrary to professional guidelines, the form at Hopkins made no mention of the specific involvement of a trainee in the procedure.

A barely legible scrawl of the word "staff" can hardly be considered full, comprehensive and specific material information.

> I hereby give my consent and authorize Doctor *Calkins/staff* of the Johns Hopkins Hospital to perform the following operation or other procedure: *Electrophysiology testing and ablation.*

One could be forgiven for thinking that since the person who proposed and explained the procedure was Hugh Calkins, and that Hugh Calkins made clear that operator experience is essential to minimize risks and insure success, and that Hugh Calkins made clear that he–Hugh Calkins–was just the experienced professional operator needed in this situation, well one could be forgiven for making the ordinary assumption that */staff* meant nurses and technicians and the like.

They give you a pager these days when they're mucking about in your loved one's innards. I suppose it's more ergodynamic than sitting in those orange plastic chairs that line the customer lounge at the local Midas Muffler shop. In any event, I was going to take full advantage. I took me down to the waterfront in Fell's Point and went to Kawasaki Sushi, at the time a great place to eat if you found yourself outside the Green Zone in east Baltimore which is the Johns Hopkins medical complex.

Mitral valve repair shouldn't take but a few hours, according to the Docs, and then she'd be up and around in no time.

In the meantime, I was going to get something to eat and pound down some SAKE. I wasn't sure if the hospital pager would reach that far, but as Kurt Vonnegut said about cheese, what could happen to Pam that hadn't happened to her already?

Chapter 12
Presentations, Papers and Posters

> "Competition for technology creates an incentive to participate in clinical research, often sponsored by industry, another potential source of revenue for individuals, departments, and hospitals. The sponsorship by industry of both formal and informal educational seminars presents potential ethical conflicts to both invited lecturers and invited audiences."

> *– Catheterization and Cardiovascular Interventions*

IT WAS A HOT NIGHT IN DIXIE for heart docs when Cardima held its annual dinner symposium during the American Heart Association's yearly meeting in Dallas in November, 1998. The company put out a press release describing the action:

> "At this meeting, their [sic] appeared to be more intensive focus than ever before on arrhythmia management, as evidenced by the number of presentations, papers and posters addressing atrial fibrillation," stated Phil Radlick, Ph.D., President and Chief Executive Officer of Cardima.

> This level of activity illustrates the significance of AF and the need for Cardima's microcatheter technology to effectively address the treatment of AF patients. Outstanding attendance, cutting-edge topics and hands-on experience with Cardima products at our Symposium demonstrates the electrophysiology community's interest in advances in dealing with this debilitating disease. The symposium began with Dr. Hugh Calkins, Johns Hopkins University, describing recent developments.

Calkins told the crowd that the Revelation was the next big thing:

He noted the need for an atrial catheter, adding a call to industry to develop one that would work properly. "There have been many attempts to make such a device," Calkins said, but "the only one still standing right now is the Cardima Revelation." He said that he was initially skeptical of the device's ability to make decent lesions. "I told them [Cardima] that I wanted to do animal studies myself," he said, adding that he was "pleasantly surprised" with the results. Getting the device into the hands of his colleagues was a difficult endeavor, Calkins said, commenting that the FDA "never makes things easy here in the U.S."

Cardima chief Phil Radlick certainly wished the FDA would make things easier, because as he worked the tables that night, smiling and shaking hands with prospective customers, his company just posted a first quarter loss of nearly $4 million.

It was perhaps this urgent financial situation that led to a bit of overstatement in their dispatch from Dallas, in which Cardima reported the results from a recently completed AF ablation feasibility study:

> "The AF ablation study consisted of 10 patients from Massachusetts General Hospital, Stanford University and Johns Hopkins University Hospital. The study resulted in no major complications and a significant improvement in 60% of patients."

FDA documents show the study in a different light, noting that it was, after all, a feasibility study, and the point was to find out if the procedure could be done without killing the patients.

So it was a success in that there were no major complications— depending on how you define the term major—but whether or not it worked was of secondary concern.

FDA records show that, as opposed to "significant improvement" in 60% of the patients, only 4 out of the ten test subjects had reported—in short term follow-up—a reduction in symptoms, with all of the patients continuing to take anti-arrhythmic drugs.

They still had no solid data to show that right-sided ablation did any good for atrial fibrillation.

It might have been impending financial collapse that led Cardima to send this enigmatic press release out to the world announcing that Ron Berger had performed an ablation at Hopkins using an unauthorized catheter:

> April 3, 1998--Cardima, Inc. (NASDAQ:CRD) today announced that the first patient in its atrial fibrillation (AF) ablation feasibility study was successfully treated last week. The patient, a 38-year-old male who had been suffering from almost daily episodes of AF for over five years, was treated and left the hospital in normal heart rhythm.
>
> Ronald D. Berger, M.D., Ph.D., a cardiac electrophysiologist at The Johns Hopkins Hospital, treated the patient using the Cardima Pathfinder AFTC ablation catheter. Dr. Berger said, "This was a highly symptomatic man who had been suffering from AF with no potential for a cure available in the near future. We were delighted to enroll him in Cardima's clinical trial and treat his AF in a minimally invasive fashion.
>
> "We had considered a highly invasive open-heart operation called the maze procedure on this patient, but felt the minimally invasive approach would be safer in this instance. Cardima's product offered the option of a catheter-based maze procedure and we are extremely pleased with the results."

There is no evidence that Ron Berger successfully treated anybody with the Cardima Pathfinder AFTC Ablation Catheter, a forerunner to the REVELATION, and Berger is probably glad that there is no evidence for such an undertaking because it would have been illegal to do so, since the FDA had not cleared that device for an ablation study.

As for the patient leaving the hospital in "normal heart rhythm," everyone leaves the hospital in normal rhythm after an ablation whether or not the procedure was successful because they are put on anti-arrhythmic drugs to suppress irregular heartbeats caused by irritation from the ablation. And it is highly doubtful that the patient would have seriously considered undergoing open-heart surgery for the maze procedure.

But whatever it was they were trying to pull, they seem to have gotten away with it.

Everybody staying at the Hyatt Regency during the American Heart Association convention got a fruit basket and a complimentary copy of the November 1998 issue of an electrophysiology journal called PACE, which contained a report by Michele Haïssaguerre suggesting that the FDA may be on to something by declining to make things easy for the likes of Hugh G. Calkins.

In Haïssaguerre's study, 45 people underwent the procedure being advocated by Cardima. Success, loosely defined as a reduction of symptoms–on or off drugs—did not last long. A year after having the procedure, 24 people felt better. After two years, the number was down to 17, a success rate of 37%, with diminishing returns expected to continue.

Chapter 13
Who's Minding the Store?

PAM AND I MOVED to Annapolis shortly after we got married so I could look for work in Washington. I had started out to be a journalist, but by the time Pam and I had gotten together, I'd sunk to working for politicians.

We'd caught the tail end of the era when Annapolis was still a relatively small town, a very pleasant place to live where waterman worked the Chesapeake Bay for crabs and oysters, and you might run into the mayor while standing in line at the post office.

I managed to get a job in DC working for a U.S. Senator and Pam began work as a nurse at the local hospital. We had a little condo, and a little boat, and on weekends we'd sail out Back Creek toward the Naval Academy or the Chesapeake Bay Bridge.

But a rapid and massive spurt of growth started in Annapolis. Anne Arundel Hospital went from being a small community affair located downtown (where you could walk to work on a nice spring day) to a giant medical center with a sprawling campus on the edge of town. In addition to handling the explosion in the local population, the new facility was picking up overflow from neighboring counties where the hospitals had been overwhelmed.

It was no longer much fun to work there if you were a nurse. Pam started spending more time filling out forms than caring for patients.

A common complaint among the nurses Pam worked with was that there was no place nearby to buy uniforms. Every time they needed a new outfit, these women had a choice between navigating inner city Baltimore or the scarier parts of Washington, DC—as if they weren't already risking their lives at work everyday.

So we spent a couple of weekends scouting out locations, and by sheer dumb luck we found a vacant store which would turn out to be ideally situated for such a purpose. All of Pam's retirement money from her years as a nurse in Florida went into the enterprise. We rented the place and purchased just enough goods to open for business. At first, we both worked the store part-time and hired helpers, but within a few years we were both able to quit our other jobs and live by working our own business. We worked a lot and we weren't getting rich, but we owned our own business. We drove nice cars and we dined out when we felt like it. We had Sushi a few times.

But now our shop was dark and closed, and worse yet, we had opened a second location, which was struggling to establish itself, and that store was closed as well.

But the bills kept coming.

Fortified by rice wine at Kawasaki Sushi I made my way back to the hospital and started making phone calls to Pam's relatives as I waited for the surgeons to announce the outcome of emergency open-heart surgery.

"How'd it go?" Pam's mother asked from Florida, on the other end of my pay phone in the Hopkins lobby. She was referring to the ablation procedure.

"Not so good," I said, and I explained about the *complication.* In the sharp intake of breath you could hear the bottom drop out. "She's OK," I said. I told her that Pam was undergoing surgery right now to repair the mitral valve. She asked if she should book a flight and come up. I said I would if I were you.

"She's having emergency open-heart surgery right now?"

"Don't worry," I told her.

Maybe I should have told her to sit tight for now. Summoning the relatives was the equivalent of breaking the fire alarm glass in case of emergency, certainly not to be done lightly.

But it was one of the things I was pondering back there at the sushi bar.

Between courses of futomaki, I kept going over the demeanor of the players involved, especially the surgeons. While they affected confidence, it was clear from watching them communicate with each other that they were far from certain they could fix Pam's broken heart in time to head off grim scenarios.

I was starting to get a bad feeling about the whole thing. It was beginning to remind me of what happened to my dad, where one bad event led to another one, and then another and it went on for weeks and then months and you dug in at each stage and looked at the bright side and hoped for the best and then one day he was dead and there was nothing.

It was during the next call that I found about the Iron Law of School Bus Driving, which is this: You never back up – NEVER.

So when the foul mouthed fishwife who lived across the street got into a Mexican standoff on a narrow road with a rookie driver from a rival company and let fly most of her repertoire in front of the kiddies, her contract with the Marlowe Brothers School Bus Company was summarily terminated– never mind that she was in the right.

Now I had someone to look after our store while the siege was on up at Hopkins. I called her Doris, and she chain smoked generic light 100's, but you could trust her to sit behind the register at the Annapolis store anyway.

Probably.

By and by Dr. David Yuh came to the waiting room. I'd never met the man before.

He said Pam had made it through O.K.

He couldn't repair her mitral valve, he had to replace that, but she'd come through it OK and I'd get to see her soon enough—and by the way, they went ahead and took out her pacemaker and all of the leads, it wasn't doing any good anyway.

Pam first made Dr. Yuh's acquaintance when he applied a bone saw to her chest. They never did shake hands. He seemed like a decent guy, friendly enough in a formal way. He said they like to get open-heart patients off the ventilator on the same day as surgery, and the patient should be out of bed by the second day. I got to see her for a few minutes.

Although they do a good job of trying to prepare you for what someone looks like just after open-heart surgery, that's really not possible.

Judging by the puffed-up head on the pillow, this person you laid eyes on just a matter of hours ago seems to have tripled in weight. The breathing tube apparatus mostly covers her lower face and her eyes dart about like those of a trapped animal.

So what do you say? Everything's OK. The worst is over. You came through it fine. You hold her hand and look into her eyes and give smooth reassurances.

Then you get back out in the hall and you exhale.

Chapter 14
Breakthrough

> "In any event, it remains increasingly critical that the practicing physician acquire and maintain an understanding of relevant first principles of Electrophysiology. Although it is exciting, it should be kept in mind that the technology facilitates the application of those fundamental principles of Electrophysiology only for the benefit of arrhythmia patients."
>
> *– American College of Cardiology*

PROFESSOR CALKINS was browsing through the journal headlines one day in 2000, maybe cooling his heels outside the office of an executive at TASER Inc., when he saw that Haïssaguerre had struck again. Dr. Michele Haïssaguerre, the ablation pioneer from Bordeaux who'd developed the Lasso mapping catheter for Johnson & Johnson, had just published a paper about the recent discoveries he'd made with his newly patented device:

"EP Breakthroughs from the
Left Atrium to the Pulmonary Veins"

While the title of the article captures the tempo of the times, it is actually technical in nature, referring to impulses that break through established circuits and cause the electrical chaos that makes the heart quiver. Life in the EP laboratory was certainly more exciting these days because of the quest for an Afib cure. The simpler arrhythmias could, by and large, be fixed by burning a scar in a specific area inside the heart that was universal to all; the mitral isthmus, for example, or the atrioventricular junction.

But, as Calkins is fond of pointing out, Afib "is very much a moving target." They were playing electrical whack-a-mole inside the heart, using zapping catheters to make scars here and there.

Haïssaguerre had let the air out of the right-sided ablation theory in 1998 by identifying the left atrium as the likely Afib source. His new discovery further narrowed the target area to "breakthrough" points in the entrances to the pulmonary veins, which he had discovered with his new Lasso Mapping Catheter.

So, at the dawn of the new century, Hugh Calkins found himself leapfrogged by the French. Of course, among the many distinctions between Bordeaux and Baltimore was the authority of the United States Food and Drug Administration. New theories and equipment were being developed and deployed much faster than any U.S. government agency could—or maybe should—react.

Devices in Europe are approved based on whether a contraption works, if it does what it is designed to do. It's an engineering question, and they leave the medical questions to the medical community. The FDA requires proof that a device is safe and effective for a specific malady. If so, it is labeled for that specific purpose.

"One can easily see how this can increase the number of approvals needed if the manufacturer needs a separate review for each proposed disease," writes Robert J. Klepinski, in the *Journal of Medical Device Regulation*. "The speed at which devices are marketed under the procedure in Europe compared to the US approval system is largely because a device in the US is a much more complicated thing, tied up in specific disease therapy rather than standing alone."

While Johnson & Johnson's Lasso project was approved and progressing nicely in Europe, Calkins was still working to get the REVELATION sanctioned by the FDA as safe and effective system for right-sided ablations, despite the fact that he himself had all but abandoned the idea.

Citing data from 1998, Calkins would later write in a text book that "Although linear ablation confined to the right atrium to cure AF is attractive from a technical and safety standpoint, multiple trials with intermediate and long term follow up have shown it to be a largely ineffective procedure."

The thinking at Cardima, apparently, was that if Calkins could get the REVELATION approved for the right side, doctors would then be able to use it off-label for the left-side, the direction in which market was headed.

In fact, Cardima had just announced another milestone on the road to futility (and potential profitability) by releasing news that Professor Calkins had used the REVELATION system to perform a right-sided catheter ablation on an elderly woman– and nothing happened:

> *PRNewswire* October 6, 2000 – Cardima, Inc., (Nasdaq: CRDM) announced today it has treated the first patient in Phase III of its atrial fibrillation clinical trial. Dr. Hugh Calkins of the Johns Hopkins Hospital treated the patient.
>
> "The patient was a 68-year-old female with a 10 year history of paroxysmal AF," stated Dr. Calkins. "We treated her with the Revelation Tx and Cardima's new NavAblator catheters. The patient tolerated the procedure well and she has returned to work. I am very pleased with the outcome of this case and the performance of Cardima's products."

That the woman lived to see another day at work was a pleasing outcome, not because she was healed, but because it sounded like medical progress. Close enough for a press release anyway.

There was nothing in the release about how Hugh Calkins dealt with the question that Mike Ross posed in the Grand Ballroom in Gaithersburg two years earlier:

"How do you consent a patient for a right-sided-only procedure and is it ethical to do? How do we go to these patients and tell them we are going to do a procedure on the right side that it is probably not going to work, but we just need to get this data?"

Maybe Hugh Calkins told the old gal the truth: The company had too much invested to just walk away.

What Hugh Calkins told Pam in 2000 after she took his hand and placed it under her blouse was that he had never felt anything like *that* before. He was talking about being able to feel the thumping ribcage caused by the pacemaker wire that was zapping her chest wall muscles.

Calkins recorded the reason for Pam's visit that day was to get a "second opinion regarding management of pacemaker lead malfunction." That's why she was there, because after nearly two years of adjusting settings and taking various types of drugs in different combinations and strengths, she couldn't take it anymore and we wanted something done. The doctor's exclamation gave Pam some measure of satisfaction. She had at last convinced a cardiologist that, yes, she had been right all along.

Even then, when it came to the official record, Calkins noted that "the symptoms of the *pacemaker lead malfunction* became more severe when she takes her anti-arrhythmic drugs."

Actually, the pacemaker lead was functioning exactly as designed. The problem was that Dr. Grant Simons had driven it through her heart wall. But to plainly state the facts in the record would go against the physicians' code, so *pacemaker lead malfunction* it was. And he wouldn't even call it a perforation; it was more like a *partial perf,* a *microperf.*

What Calkins did about it was to turn the settings on the pacemaker so low that it might as well have been turned off. There was no significant talk about ablation that day. After all, there were plenty of notes in Pam's records indicating that she hadn't really failed anti-arrhythmic drugs.

That same week, at Biosense Webster's corporate offices in the former walnut groves of Diamond Bar, California, Maria D. Ochoa got the FedEx Letter she'd been waiting for.

Ochoa was the company's Regulatory Affairs Specialist who had been working to get Haïsseguerre's new Lasso catheter approved for use in the U.S., and in August of 2000, she got the green light in the form of a 510k letter from the FDA. With a 510k letter, Biosense Webster avoided the regulatory roadblocks that Cardima was facing with the REVELATION. They didn't need to conduct clinical trials to prove that the Lasso was safe and effective because, except for a few minor improvements, the company claimed that the Lasso was essentially the same as the mapping catheter that came before it, which the FDA had approved in 1995.

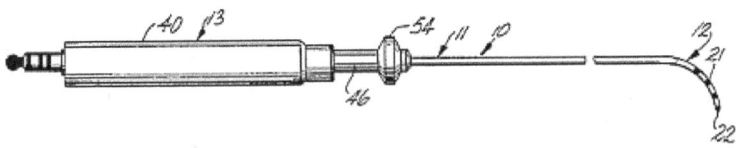

The 1995 approval of the T20 catheter was also accomplished via 510k, the manufacturer telling the FDA that, except for a few minor improvements, it was essentially the same as *its* predicate device, the "standard Cordis Webster Diagnostic 7F Deflectable Catheter" –and so on, ceaselessly into the past.

The original T20 was designed and manufactured by Webster Laboratories, before it was bought by the Cordis Corporation and became the Cordis/Webster Corporation, which was then bought by the Biosense Corporation and became Biosense Webster Inc., which was then bought by Johnson & Johnson Inc.

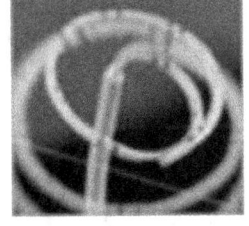

"The theory at the time was that existing lower risk devices were not a problem, and that not only could they stay on the market, but that others could emulate them," writes industry observer Klepinski. "One could compare a new product to one legally on the market, and the FDA's job is to confirm substantial equivalence."

In this way, technology has marched on, with the FDA approving new devices as substantially equivalent even though they look very different to the casual observer."

You would have to be a very casual observer indeed to not notice the difference between the original, designed by Wild Bill Webster, Caltech '49 (*Veritas Liberabit Vos*) and the one that Richard C. Wu beheld for the first time on the morning of March 25th, 2002, prior to Pam's ablation.

As Johnson & Johnson proudly points out in their 2000 application for approval, "The Lasso Mapping Catheter is substantially equivalent to the predicate devices–with the addition of the Nitinol formed 'Lasso' assembly. The platinum ring electrodes are located on the lasso assembly rather than on the catheter tip..."

So, it's pretty much the same, but it's different. Like the last one and the one before that ...

But Hugh Calkins later laid the blame for what happened to Pam on the Nitinol-formed lasso assembly. "The circular spine of our catheter became entangled in the chordae tendineae. The design, relative stiffness, and entrapment of the preformed circular spine in the mitral apparatus prevented complete straightening or relaxation of the circular tip. We suspect that the abrasive nature of the 20 electrodes caused resistance, which contributed to the inability of the catheter to slide off the mitral valve apparatus."

In fact, the Nitinol-formed lasso assembly which was spared regulatory scrutiny–on the manufacturer's say so–has gotten tangled in so many mitral valves since Dr. Richard Wu helped pioneer the technique that doctors at Harvard would publish a paper about how to deal with such a *complication* in 2004.

Chapter 15

Do we know what we're doing?

> "I think all of us are aware of the fact that the published literature probably tremendously overestimates the true efficacy of catheter ablation... "
>
> *– Hugh Calkins*

PULMONARY VEIN ABLATION for Atrial Fibrillation was all the rage there for a while, according to Hugh Calkins. "For centers that wanted to be doing the ultimate novel unknown thing," he said, "the latest thing is ablation of pulmonary veins. So the patients would be steered to that so they could build up their experience with that procedure."

Not everyone was thrilled that patients were being "steered to" having "the ultimate novel unknown thing" so that electrophysiologists could build up their experience and tell colleagues at cocktail parties that they were *au courant.*

Dr. Cox, for one, was bemused that the EP world had adopted and adapted his maze procedure. The normal disdain that surgeons generally harbor toward lesser medical professionals notwithstanding, Cox thought that the electrophysiologists' reach had certainly exceeded their grasp this time. "It is important to remember that there is such a thing as surgical precision," he writes. "When we surgeons report our results for pulmonary vein ablation, we are reporting the effects of placing a precise line of ablation around the pulmonary vein orifices. No such precision exists when cardiologists encircle the pulmonary veins with a catheter."

In adapting the Maze procedure for their catheter techniques, the cardiologists had been kind of feeling their way along, seeing what worked and what didn't work.

When it came to complications, for instance, doctors could sometimes detect pulmonary vein stenosis immediately or fairly soon after an ablation, but initially didn't think much of it:

"Focal PV stenosis is observed frequently after RF catheter ablation applied within the vein, but usually is without clinical significance," noted a 2001 study.

Not to worry.

But as the months and years went by, the stenosis got worse and the pulmonary veins were closing down. People started showing up at the doctor's office with flu-like symptoms. So the general practitioners, not privy to the inner workings of the ablationist movement, would send the patient home with some cough syrup. Meanwhile the stenosis got worse.

"A typical case is someone who had pulmonary vein ablation shows up in the ER with three pulmonary veins completely blocked and the fourth one 90% blocked," Calkins relates. "The patient gets emergency heart surgery and dies. Another person gets an Afib ablation, you get a call, the patient has been diagnosed with lung cancer, well it wasn't lung cancer, it was an occluded pulmonary vein that appeared to be lung cancer, but the patient got a lung removed," he said. "So there was this iatrogenic epidemic of pulmonary vein stenosis…"

"What we've learned obviously as we look back," he went on, "is that years ago we were ablating deep into the pulmonary veins creating all this pulmonary vein stenosis thinking we were doing good. At the end of the day, a lot of people were stepping back and saying 'We have to be out of the pulmonary veins…' "

Another lesson learned.

And the complications kept on coming, each one unexpected, and each one unprecedented. There were four reported cases of "gastric hypomotility and pyloric spasm." The victims suffered terrible bloating of their stomach and vicious bouts of vomiting because their stomachs had become permanently paralyzed.

"Just another risk to put on the consent form," said Hugh Calkins.

He wrote in 2006 about what was "perhaps the most feared and most lethal of the many complications," the atrio-esophageal fistula. They probably call it *The Widow Maker* back in the doctor's lounge. "Among patients who do not exsanguinate from upper gastrointestinal tract bleeding," a surgeon writes, "presentation includes sepsis and embolic cerebrovascular disease."

That is to say that they've burned a hole through your heart into your esophagus and if you don't drown in your own blood right then and there, you'll die very soon in some equally grisly manner.

Also, everybody in the business knows that patient injuries— *complications*—are under reported.

It was of little comfort to those who suffered the effects of these latest "previously unreported complications" that their misery added to the EP learning curve and advanced the cause of science. These patients put their very lives into the hands of physicians who led them to believe that they knew what they were doing. They trusted and believed that the doctor was looking out for them. The truth is that the doctors were learning as they went along and they obviously did not know what they were doing. They did not know the consequences of their actions.

Writing in the journal Europace in 2008, two doctors ask: "Catheter Ablation of Atrial Fibrillation: Do we know what we are doing?"

The question is the answer.

As Hugh Calkins said, nobody ever died from Afib. But many people have died from cardiac catheter ablation procedures.

With ablation in the pulmonary veins turning out to be not such a good idea, the next new thing was to ablate neat and precise lines near the entrance to the pulmonary veins.

But neatness and precision would be quite a feat, given that a catheter operator has to maneuver tiny wires around in a beating heart. First off, you've got to be able to see what you're doing, or as Calkins puts it, "Visualization of the catheter tip in relation to the cardiac anatomy is crucial."

Unlike Dr. Cox, who has no trouble visualizing his scalpel in relation to the heart because he can see them both right there with his own eyes, cardiologists like Hugh Calkins were using fluoroscopy (X-rays) to get an idea of where the catheter wires might be.

What they would do was beam X-rays through you from two different angles, and in that way, Calkins reported, "The position of the catheter in three-dimensional space can be inferred."

"In some ways, EPs are operating blind," writes Michael O'Riordan of TheHeart.org, who interviewed Dr. Mitchell Faddis of Washington University School of Medicine in St Louis for the industry's online newsletter heart*wire*:

> "It is essentially impossible to predict by X-ray where the catheter needs to be," said Faddis. "Part of the issue is being able to see the anatomy of the heart clearly in three-dimensional space and know that the catheter is sitting in the right place. Another issue is that we're moving the catheter by hand, and that's a very empiric thing.
> "We're looking at the X-ray and we're guessing that the catheter moved, but the heart's in motion the whole time.
> "With practice, you develop a sense for tiny movements, but it is still fairly indistinct."

Calkins readily acknowledges the drawbacks of using X-ray vision to make educated guesses as to the whereabouts of a medical instrument inside a beating heart.

"Another potential but less easily recognized complication associated with ablation for atrial fibrillation results from the delayed effects of radiation received by patients due to prolonged fluoroscopy times," he said.

"These risks include acute and sub acute skin injury as well as radiation-induced cancer and genetic abnormalities," he said, noting that the type of X-ray used in ablation procedures "have low penetrating power, resulting in the delivery of the maximum dose of radiation at the skin surface."

As with catheter entrapment in the mitral valve, he learned about radiation burns the hard way. He performed an ablation on a woman who came back to the hospital a month later "with acute radiation dermatitis" on her back. The patient received 400 times as much radiation during the course of the procedure than a person should absorb in a year.

"The exposure will result in an increase in her lifelong risk of skin and lung cancer," Calkins said. He blamed it on a broken switch on the X-ray machine.

And he recognized the Pin the Tail on the Donkey aspect of the whole thing: "Ablation under X-ray can be arduous," he reports, because "fluoroscopy provides only limited information about the relationship between catheter positions..."

He might as well have been using those X-ray glasses that boys ordered from the backs of comic books so they could see girls in their underwear, because as I recall, those things didn't yield any detailed anatomic information either.

Dr. Cox says that he performed the Maze procedure on about three dozen people who had undergone failed catheter ablation procedures.

He got to look inside these people's hearts and see first-hand the results of the electrophysiologists' handiwork: (And note that Dr. Cox does not recognize the self-designated subspecies electrophysiologist. They are all cardiologists to him.)

> "Their patients are not receiving a simple pulmonary vein isolation procedure as one would commonly envision that operation, but rather virtually the entire inside of the patient's left atrium is being obliterated. This is an entirely different interventional procedure....

> "Unfortunately, the patients who are undergoing this procedure by cardiologists are almost certainly unaware of the level of destruction that is being created inside their left atria and that the lesions there bear no resemblance whatsoever to a simple line of scar around the pulmonary veins. Ideally, the interventional cardiologists performing these procedures are unaware of this fact as well."

Patients undergoing catheter ablation for Afib are unaware that contrary to receiving strategically targeted and precisely placed lines of scar tissue, the insides of their hearts are actually being subjected to massive, wanton destruction—obliteration.

And Dr. Cox wants to believe that the cardiologists don't know the damage they are doing.

I am a 35 year old male who was on the VERY active side 6 months ago. I had an episode of Afib while playing basketball and in the ambulance my pulse was irregular and at 300. It was diagnosed as atrial fib.

My cardiologist recommended ablation. I had my ablation on June 21st. Since then, I have never really felt "good". Over the past 4 months, I was noticeably getting more fatigued and short of breath. A month ago, I was diagnosed with double pneumonia and was given Levaquin, 2 Z-Packs, and 3 shots of Rocephen. Nothing changed.

As a result of a right heart cath. study, and later a Pulmonary CT, I have now been diagnosed as having 2 pulmonary veins with severe stenosis and one with mild to moderate stenosis. I also have a bit of fluid in my lungs. I am currently waiting to hear from the Mayo Clinic in Rochester, MN so they can do a pulmonary vein angio/stent procedure. Have any of you heard of this complication? I have not really heard anything regarding my future prognosis yet...any clues? Needless to say, I have never been more physically and mentally down in my life!

Some cardiologists were fully aware of what Dr. Cox described as "the level of destruction created in a patient's left atria."

At the FDA's REVELATION meeting, Dr. David Schwartzman remarked about healing times after ablations. "If you watch what is happening to the atria when you ablate the bejeezus out of them, which is what we are doing, they swell like crazy," he said.

And Hugh Calkins told the same group in his role as Cardima pitchman that his experience was that "We commonly saw what looks like a gunshot blast where you have one lesion here, one lesion here, one lesion here, one lesion here, nothing continuous or linear about it." he said. "Whether these lesions are in fact pro-rhythmic, anti-arrhythmic, who really knows... this new catheter would be more doing what we are trying to do which is not ablate the atrium but put road blocks up to ablate atrial fibrillation." Hugh Calkins was trying to sell the FDA on Cardima's new catheter on the grounds that it would help cardiologists not obliterate the inside of the left atrium.

"With some of these approaches you really wonder if there's an atrium cell left at the end of the procedure," Calkins told colleagues at a dinner symposium.

Imprecise, blundering obliteration may have been what he was practicing, but it's not what he was selling. It's not the picture he presented for public consumption. It's not what the David Erdmans of the world were told–because, how else would you learn?

One has to wonder about the motivation for the duality in Calkins's portrayals of the procedure to his different audiences.

Two of his public pronouncements in 2006 illustrate the contrast between selling to perspective research subjects (patients) and reporting to colleagues.

In "The Arrival of AFIB Ablation" on the Hopkins website, the good news is delivered to Afib suffers that their worries are practically over:

Dr. Calkins "delivers radiofrequency energy around the outside of the pulmonary vessels to knock out the source of the aberrant electrical signal. Afib episodes may still occur for a few weeks, but most patients are free of them within a month."

Free at last! Thanks Doc!

But Professor Calkins has more sobering news for fellow researchers in a Cardiosource journal article that came out at the same time:

"Hugh Calkins, MD, FACC, recently co-authored a worldwide survey on the methods, efficacy, and safety of catheter ablation procedures for AF... (Only) 52.0% of catheter ablations proved "curative"... Also, it should be noted, 24.3% of patients required a second ablation procedure... The overall incidence of major complications was 6.0%, which the authors noted "is not trivial." Complications included ...death, tamponade, aortic dissection, stroke, and PV stenosis. Further, Calkins says, "We really do not have a true handle on the long-term efficacy of this procedure. Also, I personally have a problem with physicians who make the statement that their patient's atrial fibrillation is cured by catheter ablation. We really don't have data to support that claim." (The six percent complication rate referred to the overall world wide survey. The complication rate Calkins reported for his team at Hopkins was closer to 13 percent.)

In another illustration of the difference in the two faces put on the procedure is that generally, when Hugh Calkins talks about having to repeat the entire process because it failed the first time, he'll tell his peers that the patient needs a second procedure, a third procedure.

When patients complain to Hugh Calkins that the procedure didn't work, he reassures them that all they need is a "touch-up."

Why the different language—and false representation of safety and efficacy—for patients? Because he would be hard pressed to find people who would consent if they knew the danger to which they were exposing themselves by undergoing an investigational procedure at a teaching hospital.

Calkins laid it out in a breezy after dinner speech to industry insiders.

"And so we said let's take a harsh look at our numbers and see how we really did, and it was somewhat appalling. I think our success rate was about 35% for a twelve-month single procedure success rate, with a 7% complication rate. And my colleague Ron Berger says, he says, well you can't publish these data, we'll never see another patient again at Hopkins."

An appreciative chuckle rippled through the breakfast crowd.

In 2007, with his patient recruitment piece promising a safe and effective cure still displayed on the Hopkins site, he wrote an opinion piece for the journal Nature, in which he recommended that catheter ablation for Afib should not be considered as a first line therapy.

He begins by repeating what he told the FDA four years earlier, that "The true efficacy of Afib ablation remains unknown."

I don't know about the rest of the hundreds, perhaps thousands of other patients that Hugh Calkins "steered toward" what he called "the most dangerous procedure that electrophysiologists do," but he most definitely did not tell Pam and me that he thought of it as experimental procedure, that he had no idea whether the procedure actually worked, that he did not know what the risks were–and that in fact Pam would be used in a study to find those things out.

Calkins went on to say in the Nature piece that "serious complications continue to occur even in the most experienced hands... New, devastating complications are emerging, being 'discovered' on a regular basis..."

"Some doctors are pretty enthusiastic about ablation as a primary therapy," Calkins says, "but they're only enthusiastic until a patient has a stroke or some type of devastating consequence. Then the enthusiasm tends to go down a little bit."

Ah, the learning curve.

Chapter 16

The Ideal Candidate

"There are many areas in which there can be a conflict between the patient's best interest and the physician's own personal interest. The economic impact of invasive and interventional cardiology has led to pressures from several directions. Seeking increased revenues, hospitals and departments of medicine exert pressure on cardiologists for more procedures and higher fees. National and state credentialing standards for minimal procedural volumes influence cardiologists in case selection, especially low-risk cases"

– Catheterization and Cardiovascular Interventions

RESEARCH DOCTORS RECRUIT PEOPLE for clinical trials and prospective studies by putting the word out to local specialists that they are in the market for patients seeking treatment for a particular condition.

If you are a research doctor in the employ of a global corporation that pays you to train other doctors how to use certain medical devices, which they manufacture, the last thing you want is to be treating really sick people. The old and feeble are generally not resilient enough. In order to maintain high volume and foster attractive success rates, you need a hardier breed of customer; the younger and healthier, the better.

The ideal candidate for pulmonary vein ablation for atrial fibrillation is a relatively young, otherwise healthy person with occasional Afib who has failed at least two anti-arrhythmic drugs. At their first meeting, Pam was 47, otherwise very healthy, and the spin that Hugh Calkins would put on her case was that she had failed three anti-arrhythmic drugs.

So she fit the low-risk profile when her local cardiologist, who would later join the staff at Hopkins, suggested that Pam go to Johns Hopkins because they just might be able to cure her Afib.

When Pam and I drove up to Hopkins for her appointment with Hugh Calkins that September of 2001, the pall of 9/11 still blanketed the country. People went about their business, but the shock was still there, undercurrent in all conversation. There was a computer screen on his desk. The screen saver was a beautiful photograph of the original hospital. But the image was refreshed by disintegrating, which was very disturbing. Every minute or so the dome of the building, and then the brick facade, would fragment. The building would break into little pieces and collapse and disappear.

Pam saw it too and then Calkins saw it. "Guess I ought to change that," he said.

There was not much to the physical exam, since Pam's heart was strong and healthy, and for the moment, ticking away as steadily as a contented Rolex. As we perused patronizing brochures, Calkins talked about the possibility of fixing Pam's bouts of atrial fibrillation with a catheter ablation procedure.

While it was a relatively new procedure, Calkins said, he had performed it many times at Hopkins with no complications. He told us the procedure was successful in curing Afib between 80 and 85% of the time, and that if, for some reason, the procedure didn't take, she could always come back for a "touch up." There were risks as there were in any medical procedure.

The distinct take home message here was that this was an established, safe and effective procedure. You can trust me with your life, said Hugh Calkins, the Doctor of Medicine. Hugh Calkins the Research Scientist held a somewhat different view.

Somewhere in the stacks of medical journals in his office that day, there was a recent issue of *Cardiology in Review* with a paper that he wrote sizing up the state of affairs at the time.

He had concluded that "catheter ablation of AF should be considered to be an experimental procedure." The little evidence that had been collected indicated that while right-sided linear ablations may have been safe, they were not especially effective. The treatment he was proposing to Pam, pulmonary vein ablation in the left atrium, was fraught with unknown dangers to the patient but showed promise of being effective.

But the whole concept was so new that there were still a lot of unknowns. No one knew how long the effects would last. No one knew all of the side effects or complications. No one knew as yet whether the benefits of the procedure outweighed the risks to the patient.

The specific reason Hugh Calkins considered catheter ablation for Afib to be an experimental procedure in 2001 was because there were no "prospective multi-center reports to describe the results and complications."

So that's what he was doing. Although we didn't know it, the reason that Pam was in Hugh Calkins's office that day was because he had a study in progress, a study that would describe the results and complications of pulmonary vein ablation for atrial fibrillation, an experimental procedure—and she was just the kind of patient he was looking for.

Chapter 17
Stabbing Back Pains

I HAD BEEN EXPECTING Pam to be awake. I was in her room one morning after mitral valve surgery. They'd gotten her off the ventilator some time in the middle of the night. The nurse was gathering her notes and getting ready to write report, finishing up an 11p-7a shift caring for four patients. I asked her how Pam did during the night.

"Well, she was restless all night, kept twisting and moving around. Seems like she couldn't get comfortable." She lightly stroked Pam's cheek with the back of her hand. "Poor thing."

This is what she'd just written in her notes:

"Nurse's note 06:20 Pt more restless and moving constantly in bed. Has received Ativan and Fentanyl... She is reporting stabbing back pains... she has repositioned herself repeatedly..."

The nurse and I were standing on the same side of the bed facing the open door.

An unshaven young man in rumpled scrubs walked in and, without looking at us, put his hands under the sheets covering Pam's upper abdomen. The nurse and I looked at each other.

"Excuse me," said the nurse.

The intruder paid no attention and kept rooting around under the sheets. I said *Hey* and he kept going and I said *HEY* again, loudly and sharply, and that got his attention and he looked up.

The nurse and I both said: "Who are you?" He said he was from Cardiology and he was there to check on Pam's pacemaker. Then he disappeared. The nurse said she'd never seen him before.

She shrugged and went out.

Stabbing back pains... I adjusted the pillow beneath Pam's head. I slid my hand under her back to smooth out the sheet.

I felt something and pulled from beneath her lower back a pair of curved forceps.

After turning in the forceps at the nurse's station, I went to the airport to pick up Pam's mother, Jackie, who is a practical person, especially in a pinch. The women in her family would not abide incompetence in a man—husbands specifically. At the time, this did not apply to doctors. She was at the curb with her carry-on bag and got in the car as soon as I pulled up. I was able to report that Pam's heart surgery had gone well and that she was off the ventilator and in a private room.

Jackie listened to me and did not ask questions until I was through, and when her questions were answered she went silent. I was glad that she had come. She had an innate sense of how to manage a crisis. After a few days we could take Pam home and her mother could look after her while I got back to business. Everything was going to be O.K.

I told Jackie that Pam had been asleep in her room when I left, but most likely she would be sitting up in a chair beside the bed when we got there—and she could talk to us. I showed Jackie the picture in the brochure.

We entered Pam's room expecting that picture to materialize. But she was not there. The sight of the empty bed was jarring, but before I could speak a nurse came in and said that Pam had been sent back to intensive care, was back on the ventilator, and that they would tell us more when we got there.

Back up to the fifth floor.

The good news from the ICU was that Pam's temporary pacemaker, the one the mystery man from cardiology had been checking on, was in fine working order.

They could tell because when they turned it off, Pam's heart didn't work at all and the cardiac monitor showed flat lines. When they plugged it back in, the lines on the monitor resumed the rhythmic blips that normally produce the soothing lub dub, lub dub sounds of a human heart.

From now on, of course, any infant that Pam held close would hear the metallic sound of modern high technology. *Click click... Click click... Click click...* the distinct audio signature of a sturdy St. Jude Medical Model MEC-102 27mm Mechanical Heart Valve made of pyrolytic carbon and tungsten.

It's supposed to last forever.

As for why she had landed back in intensive care, extubation can be a hit or miss procedure if you're not careful. A machine has been doing your breathing for you, and getting your lungs to take responsibility again is sort of like pulling the old tablecloth trick. They've got to make sure that blood gasses are high enough so that the pump is primed and the lungs will gradually take over from the machine.

A patient must be carefully and deliberately weaned off the ventilator. It's a delicate maneuver that must be performed with care and precision.

> *Respiratory therapy note:*
>
> 22:59 Pt was extubated... Was extremely anxious and was extubated per order before mechanic or CPAP gas was up... Acute confusion and anxiety increasing...
>
> 02:01 Re-intubation performed by Anesthesia resident...
>
> 03:37 ETT position migrated. Cuff above vocal cords. Significant air leak heard. 02 sat decreasing. Ambu bag used for ventilation...
>
> 04:59 Bleeding noted on pt. gown in mid ABD area...

So they took her breathing tube out before she was ready, put the tube back in, but it came out again and started leaking so that they had to ventilate her by hand with and Ambu bag, which is sort of like a bellows, and she was a bloody mess by the time they had finally stabilized her, pulling her back from the brink once again.

And as for why her heart was not beating on its own anymore, it could be just normal, temporary post-op irritation. Or it could be that the circuit board of her heart had been accidentally blown, fried, toasted, in which case a permanent pacemaker becomes another souvenir from Johns Hopkins, like the St. Jude Mechanical Heart Valve and the attending scar tissue. For the second time in her two days in the care of Johns Hopkins Medicine, Pam's life was in free fall.

Of course, I didn't know any of this at the time. I'd been reassuring myself by reading the posters in the hall proclaiming Hopkins to be the best hospital in the land.

You cannot compare the crooks that steal your money to the ones that steal your life. I now have 2 of my 4 pulmonary veins occluded from scarring, a very disappointing cardiogram, totally disabled and hardly able to walk.

Before the operation I had a structurally sound heart with a decent electrocardiogram, except for the PVC's every minute or so. I had a benign 'lone atrial fibrillation'. If I would have been informed about the dangers of the procedure or told that the equipment was not FDA approved, I never would have elected for it.

Chapter 18

Room for Improvement

> "In this study, we provide analysis of AF ablation complications for 641 consecutive procedures. The patient population was comprised all [sic] patients undergoing catheter ablation for AF at Johns Hopkins Hospital between February, 2001 and June, 2007."
>
> *- Hugh Calkins*

OVER A SIX YEAR PERIOD beginning in 2001, at least five hundred and seventeen people underwent catheter ablations for atrial fibrillation at Johns Hopkins in order to determine the risks and benefits of pulmonary vein ablation and to evaluate newly developed techniques and equipment—and in order to train doctors to become specialists in the field.

When, upon admittance to the hospital, a person held out their left arm for the wristband to be snapped on, they got catalogued and indexed. The bar code on that wristband gave up a lot of data besides ID and blood type:

Patients were enrolled prospectively in a longitudinal patient database. Initial patient characteristics (age, gender, comorbidities including hypertension and diabetes, ejection fraction [EF], history of antiarrhythmic drug use, and cardioversions, AF subtype [paroxysmal vs persistent]) and procedural data (ablation strategy, case duration, transseptal access duration, operator) were systematically recorded.

In the initial series of studies, there would be three ablation strategies. The first 75 people would be treated with the approach Haïsseguerre developed in Bordeaux, in which scars were burned into segments of tissue outside the entrance to the pulmonary veins. The next 75 patients would be steered toward the circumferential or "Pappone approach," which burned a continuous circular scar, then another 70 or so people would get a combination of the two approaches, and so on...

Calkins knew that the complication rates would be highest among the earliest patients to have each procedure because no one had experience with these particular techniques and catheters. So there would be the usual learning curve until they got past the first 100 patients. Inevitably, more people would get hurt at the beginning, until operators became familiar with the tools and comfortable with the technique. The learning curve in this case would be especially hard on patients, given the physician training program under which it would be carried out.

The number of Afib ablation procedures being performed in the U.S. saw a big increase in 2001 as medical research centers began gearing up studies to evaluate the new concepts developed in Europe.

Calkins kicked off his ambitious study project with a pulmonary vein ablation performed in February, 2001.

A few heady weeks later, the first report came in to MAUDE, the FDA's Manufacturer and User Facility Device Experience Database, about a Lasso catheter getting caught in a mitral valve.

> *Adverse Event Description: Physician inadvertently guided the catheter into the left ventricle. The catheter tip was caught in the mitral valve during an attempt to pull catheter into the left atrium... the circular tip of the catheter detached from its transition area and the tip subsequently migrated into the aorta descendens...*

There is no way to tell from the report at which hospital this occurred or how the patient ultimately fared after having a metal shaving let loose in his descending aorta.

This was the first of many adverse event reports to come as the procedure became more widely practiced. Eventually, *Circular Mapping Catheter Entrapment in the Mitral Valve Apparatus* would become known as a signature *complication* of pulmonary vein ablation for atrial fibrillation, along with stroke, pulmonary vein stenosis and a host of other procedure-related disasters.

They discovered the risks of the procedure—and the dangerous aspects of the devices—as reports began to come in from the field, reports that Johnson and Johnson used to refine its product.

The paper that Calkins published about Pam's *complication* contained recommendations, written for the benefit of J&J engineers in New Brunswick, as to how to improve the catheter design.

Calkins may believe that Johnson & Johnson pays him because they want to help him relieve suffering and cure a difficult disorder.

But at bottom, he is being paid by a device manufacturer to field test a product and report the results. And as reports started coming in, it became apparent that there were certainly some kinks, so to speak, to be worked out with the Biosense Webster Lasso Mapping Catheter:

The nature of the reports suggests a typical design evolution in which earlier products may show some room for process improvements and, once addressed, those complaints diminish.

There were so many casualty reports coming in as the procedure became more widespread that some in the EP community began to publish their concern that things were getting out of hand in the catheter ablation technology sweepstakes:

"The tip of the lasso catheter broke off. The procedure was aborted when the catheter fractured. Upon removal of all catheters and sheath a tiny piece of mitral tissue was attached to the broken point of the Lasso. A surgeon was contacted for urgent surgical removal of the catheter tip from the mitral valve..."

And: "When an audible pop was heard, physician removed the catheter from the patient and observed that the tip of the catheter had loosened from its shaft. The bond between the deflectable tip and its shaft was broken, but still held together by internal wiring. There was some evidence of insufficient polyurethane. Biosense Webster taking corrective action..."

And: "The electrode got caught on the edge of the sheath's tip causing damage and making a sharp edge on the ring... manufacturer taking action to address and resolve this issue..."

And: "It was reported that during a mapping procedure, the lasso catheter became entangled in the mitral valve. While attempting to untangle the catheter, the loop separated from the shaft. During attempts to retrieve the tip, atrial perforation occurred. The perforation could not be attributed to a specific catheter. The patient underwent surgery to remove the loop section and repair the perforation of the left atrium...:

And: "A biosense webster navistar catheter was being used in the left atrium. About 30 minutes into the procedure, the patient's blood pressure dropped. Using cardiac echo, pericardial effusion was observed. Pericardiocentesis was performed, but the patient's chest had to be opened. Patient was stabilized and taken to surgery. At the time of the drop in blood pressure, the navistar (biosense webster) catheter was being repositioned. The patient expired upon removal of life support 3 days after the procedure..."

Because of the laxity in reporting *complications* and *adverse events,* no will ever know exactly how many people were injured or had *expired* in the early phase of the industry's learning curve.

In March of 2001, Dr. Marcus Wharton at the Medical University if South Carolina posed a question in his essay "Ablation of atrial fibrillation: a procedure come of age?" His answer was that—with casualty rates approaching 25%—the coming of age was a long way off:

"It is clear from the available information that curative ablation approaches for AF are rapidly advancing, but too little is known at present to advocate widespread implementation. In particular, given the potential for serious complications, even with ablation of AF initiators in healthy individuals, it is difficult to advocate ablation as front line therapy.

"Furthermore, the procedures are technically difficult, arduous, time-consuming, and are not cost-effective. Given the risks of serious complications, even in experienced hands, a loud note of caution must be expressed concerning widespread application by individuals who are inexperienced in technical aspects of the procedure.

"More importantly, rates of major complications in the prospective studies have been unacceptably high, occurring in approximately one-quarter of patients. Although symptomatic control with continued antiarrhythmic drug therapy can be achieved in the majority of patients, the high rates of serious complications significantly limit application of these procedures to only a few, heavily symptomatic patients, and hamper enrollment of patients in studies evaluating new technologies that are aimed at simplifying the procedure.

When this paper was published, Hugh Calkins was still going through the motions of performing right-side ablations on people in order to complete the Cardima study, and Dr. Wharton agreed with Calkins' views on the merits of that exercise:

"Limitation of the linear lesions to the right atrium greatly simplifies the procedure and avoids the potential risks associated with creation of linear lesions in the left atrium. Right-atrium-only linear lesion sets rarely cure patients with paroxysmal AF, however, and are ineffective in chronic AF."

Dear Mr. Walter,

Our daughter underwent ablation procedure for atrial fibrillation at the Medical University of South Carolina on Dec. 1. The last two weeks have been our worst nightmare.

They made a puncture which they did not see. Later in a "regular" room, her heart leaked blood into the pericardium, ultimately resulting in cardiac arrest. The upshot is that her brain was deprived of blood and the essential oxygen for an undetermined length of time. Jenny has been in a coma for two weeks and EEG's show minimal brain activity. Doctors began discussing withdrawing life support as soon as day number four.

Questions: How long was your wife in the state when her heart pumped very little blood? How long was your wife in a coma? What did her EEGs indicate? Were you advised to stop life support because recovery was extremely unlikely? What brought her out of the coma? Did the doctors ever mention "anoxic brain injury"? What treatment was given your wife? (Jenny got no particular treatment, simply allowed time to pass.)

The doctor's name is Marcus Wharton. I would appreciate an early response since we face terrible decisions in the near future. We would also appreciate your prayers.

Thank you very much.

In June 2001, Cardima announced it had been awarded a patent for the REVELATION Tx, which it described as "a method of linear ablation which allows a physician to perform minimally invasive linear surgical cuts, saving cost and replacing a highly invasive, open-chest procedure.... Cardima Inc. developed the REVELATION Tx system for the treatment of AF, which the company estimates is a potential $6 billion market."

You could make a lot more than $6 billion with a minimally invasive alternative to open heart surgery if you could get people to believe you had one. Along those lines, the company announced that Phase III trials were going swimmingly, and once they were completed, it was on to the Holiday Inn at Gaithersburg.

"We are encouraged by the continued confidence and positive experience physicians participating in the Phase III study are reporting after using the REVELATION Tx to treat their patients," said CEO Gabriel Vegh, adding, with what turned out to be wild optimism, that "We are targeting FDA approval of the REVELATION Tx by the end of this year."

Seventy nine more patients would have to undergo right-sided catheter ablation procedures before Phase III clinical trials were finished for the REVELATION and Cardima could apply for approval to market the ablation system as an effective treatment for atrial fibrillation. It couldn't happen fast enough either.

The company was burning through $600,000 a month.

Chapter 19

Room 101

> **"**The patient has a right to be fully informed not only about the procedure being planned but also who specifically will be performing the procedure. If a fellow-in-training will play a major role in the procedure or if physician extenders are used, their roles and responsibilities should be explained to the patient. No matter what roles others play, the attending cardiologist is still responsible for every aspect of the procedure."
>
> *– Catheterization and Cardiovascular Interventions*

IT WAS ALMOST 7:45 AM on Monday, March 25th, 2002. Dr. Richard Chao-Chung Wu was running late, and by the time he'd made it to Lab Room 101 and scrubbed in, the patient was sedated and ready to go.

Wu got his MD at Duke in 1994, and had been at Hopkins ever since. He'd spent three years as an Internal Medicine Resident, then four years doing a Cardiovascular Disease Fellowship, and was capping off his resume with a Fellowship in Clinical Cardiac Electrophysiology. He was being mentored in the freewheeling world of electrophysiology research by Hugh Calkins, being groomed to practice and then teach catheter ablation for atrial fibrillation. His next stop would be a stint with Warren "Sonny" Jackman in Oklahoma, and then on to run his own EP Lab at a major medical center. He was on his way, a paid disciple of a procedure that was more corporate strategy than cure.

That's if he could get thirty Afib procedures under his belt. These things looked to be pretty tricky and despite all his previous experience at Hopkins, Wu was not so sure of himself that morning. Having received his assignment the night before, he had never met the patient—and with any luck, he never would.

Technically, he was supposed to meet with them before the procedure to do a physical assessment and get the informed consent signature, but who has time? As long as he'd gotten started and had the catheters in position in time for when Calkins showed up to watch him do the transeptal puncture, he'd be OK.

Under the spotlight his gloved hands opened a sterile package and he looked curiously at the sparkling Nitinol tip of a Biosense Webster Lasso Mapping Catheter.

And how do we know that Richard Wu showed up in Room One after his patient had been sedated, and therefore could not have completed his informed consent chores that morning?

For one thing, Pam's daughter and I were there with Pam that morning. Her daughter Kristi was with her right up to the minute she was wheeled into the lab. Neither Calkins nor Wu came to meet Pam beforehand.

Another indicator is that on the physical assessment sheet he was supposed to have initialed during his examination of Pam, which he would have done after he had fully informed her of the implications of what she was about to undergo, Richard Wu had to overwrite the initials of the staffer who actually did the assessment.

And Wu signed his name as the person who gave Pam informed consent at 7 AM on the morning of the procedure. I know that he signed the form after the fact, because the signature of the person who witnessed Pam's scribbling of her name and initials on all those forms belongs to me.

Chapter 20

A Dangerous Instrument

"We're missing a lot of things at this point," Dr Hugh Calkins (Johns Hopkins University Medical Center, Baltimore, MD) told heart*wire*. "Everything is based on, 'This is how I think my patients are doing.' If history holds true, the results are always worse when the procedure is held up to a multicenter, rigorous study, where you prospectively define the complications and evaluate. We need better data on the true efficacy and safety of the procedure in patients selected as part of a multicenter study in a rigorous, prospective fashion."

"Fig Newton?"

I was peeling the lid from a coffee cup. I told Pam's mother No, thanks.

We were on a bench in the hall right outside the ICU. There wasn't much to say, so we fell into a trance watching the doors on elevators open and close. Sometimes people got out, sometimes they didn't. Sometimes there were no people.

Hugh Calkins appeared, all lab coat and glasses, a contrite and timid presence.

He carried a medical instrument. He sat down next to Pam's mother, Jackie. He was terribly sorry about what happened.

He said this to her:

"What happened was I was trying to reposition the catheter. I was going to ablate four areas. I got two done and I wanted to switch catheter sheaths. I turned away for a second and the mapping catheter–just like this one here–see how it's coiled up there at the end like a Lasso? And that's what they call it, a *Lasso* catheter..."

"Well, while I was moving the catheter, working toward the third area, I turned away because I wanted to use a different sheath, and the catheter went down into the mitral valve muscles.

"The mitral valve muscles, they're like parachute strings. And you see how this catheter loop sort of coils up? When we retract it, it's supposed to straighten out and it should have just slid off those muscles when we retracted it, but this catheter, you know, is a mapping catheter, which, they have these little electrodes on them."

He held the tip of the catheter up and ran the thin wire straight through his fingertips before it snapped back to a curl. "Now this one, this mapping catheter is a new design," he said. "It has TWENTY sensors–electrodes. So what I think is... is that the extra sensors kept us from retracting the catheter. The electrodes of this catheter got snagged on these parachute string muscles of the mitral valve."

"This catheter," said Hugh Calkins, "is a dangerous instrument."

One thing I remember very clearly is that when he told me the story he said he was using a *decapolar* catheter. The word decapolar stuck in my mind. Deca, decade, ten. He told me the catheter had ten sensors.

It doesn't really matter, but we'll never know the answer because the catheter was "lost" after the procedure.

They were supposed to turn it in for an inspection after they filed an adverse event report with the FDA, but the Lasso catheter in question disappeared somewhere between Lab Room 101 and the CCU.

Yesterday, I'd felt almost sorry for Calkins. Just a decent guy, trying to do a good job. He seemed genuinely aghast and remorseful, and the younger doctor with him was noticeably shaken. You could see how much these two cared about Pam, and seeing as how she would make a nice recovery, I tried to take an expansive view of the situation.

These things happen. I remember thinking how we all take these modern medical miracles in stride, and that perhaps we had come to expect too much of the medical community.

Transplants and re-attached limbs and bypass surgery, all these things we take for granted.

But I was beginning to narrow my view now that the promised resurrection had failed. At first, I'd given Calkins credit for stepping up to the plate and taking responsibility. Whatever else, I had to admire the fact that he was being a stand-up guy.

Now I wasn't so sure. Listening to him tell the story again, I found myself wondering how a man of his experience could have made such a rookie mistake. And how was it that he was just now discovering that he had deployed a dangerous instrument?

"Let me ask you something, Doc," I said. "When you're moving the catheter around inside the heart and you want to move the Lasso part from one site to another, don't you pull the catheter back into the sheath before you move it, then let it out at the new site?" It seemed like common sense to me. Calkins pushed his thick, rimless glasses back up the bridge of his nose and nodded.

"Oh, yes" he said, "That's what we'll do from now on."And thus I made my contribution to the annals of medicine and medical device usage. In his official description of the fiasco, *Circular Mapping Catheter Entrapment in the Mitral Valve Apparatus: A Previously Unreported Complication*, published in the Journal of Cardiovascular Electrophysiology a few months after the fact, among the suggestions Calkins makes as to avoiding the disaster inflicted on Pam is this: "… it would be reasonable to withdraw the catheter into the sheath during repositioning or moving of the catheter between the inferior PVs."

If only I'd thought of that sooner.

Despite his declaration that the Lasso Catheter was a dangerous instrument, Calkins continued to endorse its use. There have been nearly 200 more reported adverse events with the Lasso catheter since. In 2008, after one too many mitral valve been lassoed, the latest model was recalled.

Around the time that Pam became one of the first 100 unwitting participants in the big Afib ablation study underway at Hopkins, two prominent *kardiologe herzspezialists* at the University of Leipzig's Department of Electrophysiology, Drs. Hindricks and Kottkamp, were writing an editorial in the Journal of Cardiovascular Electrophysiology that would have been of interest to Hugh Calkins.

For one thing, he serves as a senior editor at the journal, and the editorial, titled *Potential Benefits, Risks, and Complications of Catheter Ablation of Atrial Fibrillation: More Questions than Answers*, wonders whether Calkins may have been pushing things a bit.

They ask, "Is radiofrequency ablation for atrial fibrillation currently a procedure with an acceptable and well-balanced benefit-to-risk profile?" and, "Is it really true that radiofrequency ablation targeting pulmonary veins is an established procedure?"

They say no.

"Neither success rates nor complication rates currently [2002] are well defined," they say. "Catheter ablation procedures to cure atrial fibrillation are still in a continuing stage of development... typical complications associated with a certain procedure may occur rarely; thus, large numbers are necessary to recognize specific risks."

Of course, Calkins was doing his part to put some big numbers on the board. While the editorial was being drafted in Leipzig, he went to Milan, Italy for lunch with Dr. Carlo Pappone. There, after sampling the San Raffaele Hospital cafeteria's world famous risotto, Calkins would pick Capatto's brains about the circumferential approach, which would be tried out on the second batch of subjects back in Baltimore.

Chapter 21

It's Making Money for the Hospital

"In view of the major impact of medical economic forces, rapidly changing technology, and other pressures on invasive cardiologists, the Society for Cardiovascular Angiography and Interventions determined that a statement of the ethical issues confronting the modern invasive cardiologist was needed. The various conflicts presented to the cardiologist in his or her roles as practicing clinician, administrator of the catheterization laboratory, educator, or clinical researcher were reviewed. In all instances, the major concern was determined to be the welfare of the patient no matter how forceful the pressures from various outside force or concerns for personal advancement might be."

– Catheterization and Cardiovascular Interventions

THESE GUYS had big plans.

In a PR piece that appeared in heart*wire,* Dr. Peter Gallagher disclosed a vision that suggested he spent too much time watching *The Jetsons* when he was little. Gallagher, Gorden Tomassoni, and "Sonny" Jackman were interviewed about a catheter navigation system manufactured in a joint venture between Biosense Webster and Stereotaxis, Inc. called *Niobe.*

It was an automated system, designed to free the attending physician to deal with more pressing matters.

> Since February 2003, EPs at Lexington's Central Baptist Hospital Heart Institute have been using powerful electromagnets to guide catheters and guidewires through the heart... In Lexington, home to Gallagher and Tomassoni, the duo have begun off-label work with the Niobe system to test the effectiveness of magnetic navigation in lead implantation for biventricular pacing procedures.
>
> "Soon, we'll be able to sit down in the control room while performing several procedures," Dr Peter Gallagher, an EP at Central Baptist, explained to heart*wire*. Hinting at the possibility of one day performing many mapping and ablation procedures by remote control, Gallagher said that a day will arrive when EPs can "sit down and have their coffee" while they map and ablate some of the heart's trickiest arrhythmias.

From what I can tell, a lot of EP's are already sitting down and having their coffee while they nominally map and ablate some of the heart's trickiest arrhythmias.

The autoablator machines went for $2 million a pop.

But it's worth it, advised Jackman, you'll make your money back in no time.

Catheter ablation for Afib was the wave of the future, the bread & butter for EP Labs. He urged fellow practitioners to buy:

> "While the cost of the system may scare off some hospitals and EP labs, Jackman sees a benefit in making the investment, especially if it means being able to keep patients and not needing to refer them to high-volume specialists."

"Electrophysiology is just exploding right now. It's making money for the hospital... About 70% of patients I see are referred from other physicians, and 80% of these come from out of state," said Jackman. "They're referred because the procedures are difficult and other EPs don't want to do them."

"Or maybe because they're dangerous and they think that I could weather the storm if heart block occurred better than they could. But what if they can now do these procedures as well as I can? They may be in a small town, but they have a lot of patients. They shouldn't have to refer to me. If their hospitals buy a machine like this, they can now keep those patients and make the same profit in EP that our hospital is making. "

One possible reason for all the love was not mentioned in the article: Tomassoni, Gallagher and Jackman are on the board of directors for Stereotaxis. And Dr. Jackman has served as a paid consultant all the way back to Webster Laboratories.

Chapter 22

A Previously Unreported Complication

> **"**I always like to ask, 'Does it meet the mother test?' That is, would you want your mother to undergo such an intervention?"
>
> *- Howard Cohen, MD*

WHEN I READ Hugh G. Calkins's journal article about what happened to Pam, I thought at first that he is not a very good writer. But now, after having read it many times, I see it as a masterpiece of mind-bending logic. An article to report a previously unreported complication, which cites two previous reports of the complication being reported.

Here are two sentences in the order in which they were published in the peer-reviewed *Journal of Cardiovascular Electrophysiology* Vol. 13, No. 8, August 2002:

> "Entrapment of a circular mapping catheter in the mitral valve apparatus during focal AF ablation is a serious and previously unreported complication. A review of the literature reveals that catheter entrapment in the mitral valve apparatus has been reported in association with catheter ablation procedures."

The fact that this makes perfect sense to the author and his peers illustrates a main aspect of this story: The melding of Science, Medicine and Academia at teaching hospitals has rendered the patient an abstract part of the healing equation.

Catheter injury to a mitral valve, the *complication* that took Hugh Calkins by surprise in Pam's case, has long been recognized by the American College of Cardiology as a risk of any cardiac catheterization because it is common sense: "Certain risks are associated with RF ablation. They include the general risks of any cardiac catheterization, such as valvular damage..." Hein Wellens, 1999.

"The catheter should be carefully manipulated in order to avoid entrapment into the mitral valve apparatus." Hindricks G: *Eur Heart J* 1993. Hugh Calkins himself has written that catheter manipulation can cause valvular damage, and he should know, because he was manipulating a catheter that damaged someone's heart valve in 1991.

So why the compulsion to publish a story about a botched ablation? Especially since, according to what the attending physician told the patient and her family, the error occurred because he'd taken his eye off the ball.

Most doctors would be embarrassed. But if you are helping to field test equipment and you can present it as news, a scientific discovery, then you can add another title to your list of publications. And that's what it's all about. In order to stay on top of the field you've got to publish. The patients become statistics, they come and they go, and after a while a certain detachment begins to take hold.

Not surprisingly, an elitist attitude pervades the upper echelons at hospitals like Hopkins. As a Harvard graduate recently commented, "In medical school we were actively encouraged to be leaders in medicine, and not necessarily good doctors."

Research and academic professor/physicians are generally out to prove a theory or test a procedure or product. You are not a patient coming to get well, you are one of forty patients in a defacto medical trial. You are an endpoint for a study, a chance to try out a new technique or device.

Your body is the proving grounds for newcomers to medicine and their new hardware. Here is an extract from an editorial in the *Journal of Thoracic and Cardiovascular Surgery,* titled *Surgery as Spectacle* by Dr. Duke Cameron of Johns Hopkins. It is a thoughtful piece discussing the pros and cons of telecasting live open-heart surgery. The words in parentheses are Dr. Cameron's, in the original text.

> "Several of my colleagues have also been witness (rhymes with accomplice) to intraoperative disasters... including patient deaths in what should have been straightforward procedures... and who later confessed a sense of collective guilt and shame that discouraged them from pursuing their own experience with the new technique.

> "I once viewed a live telecast valve repair that resulted in a clearly unacceptable outcome but was tolerated because... I suspect... the surgeon did not want to publicly acknowledge failure and replace the valve."

A clearly unacceptable outcome was tolerated.

Tolerated by whom? Maybe witness doesn't really rhyme with accomplice, but the point is well taken. A witness to a crime may be inclined to report it and to help the victim. An accomplice would not. I doubt that Dr. Cameron and his colleagues confessed their complicity in these intraoperative disasters to the families of the victims. Shame and guilt will only go so far. Most likely, the attending surgeon came out shaking his/her head and explained to somebody's wife or mother or son that there had been a complication, a very rare complication.

And most likely, the stunned family member, having been trained to believe in the infallibility of medicine, a reader of *US News & World Report,* said thanks, Doc, I know you did the best you could, and they buried their loved one and tried to go on.

I find myself 48 years old and a widow because we believed the lofty promises that are not true. Peace will be a long time coming for me because both myself and my husband were lied to about this procedure. Because he was in such great physical shape (an athlete), we were led to believe that the only risks were from the anesthetic. He was well controlled on the medication, but had an ablation. So, at 53 he drove himself to the hospital.

It appears that the catheter punched a hole in his heart. Then to compound the error, it wasn't recognized soon enough and by the time they reacted, his brain was severely damaged. They brought him back (with mixed messages as to how long he was "down"), but he was dramatically brain damaged and died 8 days later. He lived for 8 agonizing days during which I was forced to make unspeakable decisions including removing him from life support.

He was an athlete who completed multiple Ironman Triathlons and was in amazing physical shape. He had a huge heart (no pun intended) and he was willing to help anyone who needed it. It was really apparent after he was gone how many lives he touched in his short time. I loved him dearly and have a hole in my own heart that will likely never heal completely.

Calkins, et al, would protest that *publishing Circular Mapping Catheter Entrapment in the Mitral Valve Apparatus: A Previously Unreported Complication* was really a selfless act designed to warn fellow practitioners of a complication heretofore unknown.

If you discount the fact that the report was basically feedback for the R&D people at J&J, Calkins's paper sent this message, more or less, out to interventional cardiologists everywhere: Attention: Keep an Eye on that Dangerous Catheter You've Let Loose in Your Patient's Beating Heart—which makes about as much sense as a safety bulletin warning about the dangers of wearing a neck tie while operating a lathe:

Necktie Entrapment While Operating a Lathe:
A Previously Unrecognized Complication
of Making a Lamp in Woodshop

We describe the entrapment of a Salvatore Ferragamo Gancini Print silk necktie secured with a simple Windsor knot within the rotational apparatus of a Ganesh GHT-59 Super-Precision Hardinge-type 2nd operation lathe (DV-59 copy) with a 3-horsepower electronic variable speed motor. A review of Popular Mechanics reveals 16 adverse outcomes last year when some portion of a lathe operator's necktie became entangled in the moving parts of a lathe.

The occurrence of this previously unreported complication involving a Salvatore Ferragamo Gancini Print silk necktie stresses the need for continual monitoring and reporting of adverse effects from new devices and procedures to better inform lathe operators as to proper neck attire.

Based on our experience, several recommendations can be made that may lower the possibility of this complication occurring in the future...

Disclosures: Dr. Calkins receives research funding from the Salvatore Ferragamo Foundation, serves as a paid consultant for Ganesh Industries, and is on the editorial board of Popular Mechanics.

Chapter 23
Just one of Those Things

THE COFFEE URNS WERE STEAMING and the Danishes were piled high. It was a little before 9am on a rainy Thursday in May, 2003. The FDA's Circulatory System Devices Panel was convening again at the Gaithersburg Holiday Inn. Professor Calkins went through his notes for the big presentation one more time. Others read the Wall Street Journal or looked through their information packets.

Calkins, taking time out from his big pulmonary vein ablation study, was there in order to persuade his friends and colleagues on the panel to approve Cardima's REVELATION Tx cardiac catheter ablation system. It was an elaborately choreographed Power Point presentation, which would work nicely in the newly renovated Walker/Whetstone Room.

On the street out front, first responders were in full swing at the scene of a gory head-on collision that tied up traffic and made a couple of sales reps from Medtronic late for the meeting. At 9:18, Chairman Warren K. Laskey, M.D. looked at his Rolex. He tapped his microphone. The doctors put their Danishes down and the meeting came to order.

Before Hugh Calkins could get in there and pitch for Cardima, there was other business to be dealt with, and pretty grim business at that. Laskey told the group that "Before we commence with the topic of the day, there will be a brief presentation by Marian Kroen of the FDA ..."

Marian had been dispatched from the Issues Management staff at the ominous-sounding Office of Surveillance and Biometrics to alert the cardiology world to a potential danger. Two people had died, or, in the parlance of the trade, there had been *adverse events* involving Medtronic products.

Medtronic makes some sophisticated gadgets. They make implantable medicine pumps, and stents for clogged arteries. They make neurostimulators, which are electrodes buried deep in the brain to help Parkinson's disease patients. For stubborn muscle pain, there is diathermy, which is basically a way to warm up your muscles via microwave.

A couple of people who had both stimulators in their brains and sore backs went to get their muscles microwaved. They fell asleep and never woke up. Medtronic and the FDA had done some tests to figure out what exactly had felled the victims, and an autopsy was performed on one of the expired medical consumers.

Conclusion: A deadly interaction of the two Medtronic devices.

It seems that sometimes the electromagnetic field from the diathermy heating pads cause the electrode tips stimulating a person's brain to turn red hot, which cooks the brain from the inside out. The good news is that because the brain has no pain receptors, the victims don't feel a thing, which I suppose would count as a victory in the eyes of the director of the pain clinic.

"So what did the FDA do?" said Marian, "We reached into our toolbox and took some actions." Bold actions. The FDA made Medtronic put bigger warning labels on the packages of both devices, so that both neurosurgeons and pain docs could beware the broiled brain.

Some of the cardiologists seemed impatient, *What's this got to do with us?*

"As you all know," said Marian, "Cardiac ablation happens at around 50 to 55 degrees Celsius... " The cardiologists did indeed know that when a wire inserted into the heart raises nearby tissue to about 130° F it kills that tissue, which creates scar tissue, which blocks the pathway of rogue electrical beats that cause your heart to quiver.

That's the idea anyway.

Her point was that there may have been adverse interactions between pacemakers, defibrillators and diathermy—as a matter of fact there should have been—but there were no reports. How can that be?

Pacemakers and defibrillators had leads, like the brain stimulators, and so there should have been reports. "There have been warning labels about pacemakers on diathermy equipment for a long time," said Marian, "but, as we all know, who reads the labeling?"

Doctors are apparently no different from husbands and fathers in their scorn for directions. Just rip open the package and start figuring it out.

After advancing various theories as to why brains were getting cooked while hearts seemingly remained unscathed, Marian invited comment from the group.

Perked up and prepared for questions, she was met with a strong showing of apathy.

Warren Laskey broke the spell. He didn't think it was a big deal. "For openers," Laskey said, "I don't know if any of it makes sense, and it's not a trivial exercise to reposition pacemaker leads. I think if it were really more than a curiosity, you would hear more about it. Do my colleagues have any thoughts?"

A cardiologist on the panel asked what it was that made some diathermy/brain patients more vulnerable to injury than others. Marian deferred to Paul Rejarica, a representative from the FDA's Office of Science and Technology, which had performed some tests.

"I don't know," he said. "It's just one of those things."

Dr. Laskey looked up and peered out over nearly invisible reading glasses. "All right, thank you. We're puzzled as well. Let's move on ..."

Interestingly, the day before Marian Kroen made her nerve-tingling presentation in Gaithersburg, two stern and professional looking businesswomen met in the parking lot of a suburban medical complex in Columbia, Maryland, along the I-295 corridor between the nation's capital and Charm City, USA.

In a classic pincer maneuver, Inspector Stephanie Shapley descended from the FDA's Baltimore District Office to the northeast, while Safety Officer Barbara Crowl moved in from the agency's Bethesda office to the southwest. Briefcases and clipboards in hand, they got out of their government vehicles, joined forces in the lobby, and mounted a surprise inspection of a company which was conducting clinical research trials in conjunction with Johns Hopkins Medicine—on implanted stimulators for chronic pain.

The study was being run by two doctors from Hopkins, neurosurgeon Richard North and his wife Catherine North, an oncologist, collectively known as North Family Inc., which begat Stimsoft, Inc., which was developing the pain stimulator technology being used in the study.

The inspection turned up a number of irregularities and violations: investigators were not following the established protocols, documentation was missing, forms not completed. The most egregious violations involved informed consent. A number of people being used for research were not informed that they were being treated with an investigational device. In some cases, consent forms were signed after the procedure was performed. In some cases the witness's signature was filled in some time after the subject had signed the consent form.

The raid could not have come at a worse time, thought the Norths, because they were trying to close a deal for the sale of their company to Medtronic, the company that was sponsoring their clinical trials.

Their arrangement with Johns Hopkins had been to develop radio frequency, or RF technology, for their stimulators. But the Norths had also developed an alternative energy system for the devices. They called their system Polaris, and they'd sunk a ton of their own money into the independent project. Medtronic, eager for their Polaris system, had agreed to buy Stimsoft from North Family Inc. for $10 million.

The threat to the deal came not from FDA warning letters about the deceit, sloppiness and other irregularities of the clinical studies. The real snag came when Johns Hopkins University President William R. Brody decided that JHU should get a piece of the action.

Terms of the sale required Hopkins to sign a release of any claims to Stimsoft intellectual property. Brody, the highest-paid university president in the United States, was on the board of directors for Medtronic. He demanded that the Norths pay JHU $1.24 million before he would sign the waiver. JHU owed the Norths $455,000 in laboratory fees, so Richard North had to mark that bill paid and write out another check for $829,000 to Hopkins Inc. before the deal could go through.

Chapter 24

CCU

WHEN IT COMES TO STRESS positions, sleep deprivation and drugs, the torture techniques we adopted from the enemy in the last war have nothing on what goes on at most modern intensive care units. Imagine being strapped to a 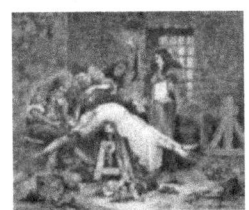 gurney, humiliated, drugged and disoriented, bright lights burning incessantly overhead, strangers sticking you with needles and shoving tubes down your throat, no food, no sleep, no water for days and days and days …

Welcome to Nelson 5 CCU at Johns Hopkins Medicine

I'm not faulting the individual doctors and nurses that work the place, but somehow a system designed to save lives and care for people evolved into a high-tech torture chamber.

Would it be so difficult to swing that spotlight over, just a bit, so the patient is not getting the 3rd degree all night long? Does the intern have to shatter the patient's exposed nerves by slamming the metal clipboard onto the bed rail when he shouts out his greetings at 2 AM? (Not that you'd know what time it was.)

Do you think maybe you could have a little sign somewhere in the patient's field of vision saying something like:

No, you're not in Hell. You're in the CCU.
Today is Tuesday, April 11, 2002.
You've been here for THREE WEEKS

Chapter 25

The Spin You Put on It

> "The process of obtaining informed consent from patients mandates and pre-supposes that physicians, first, are fully informed of the risks and benefits of the therapy that they are offering. It is ethically imperative that we are honest with the data, so that we can be honest with our patients."
>
> *- Dr. Roderick Tung*

AT THE HOLIDAY INN, Hugh Calkins found himself at the center of an EP pecking party. His premier presentation of Cardima's REVELATION catheter ablation system had not gone over well.

The chief argument he made for the REVELATION system was that it had to be better than the current alternative to the drag and burn, which was pulmonary vein isolation, the very procedure that he'd let Richard Wu practice on my wife.

Hugh Calkins told the FDA in 2003 that pulmonary vein ablation, which he was promoting and practicing at the time, was neither safe nor sound. At the same time that he was recruiting patients for the procedure on his website, advertising a proven and effective therapy that cured Dave Erdman the mountain climber, he was telling government regulators that "the safety and efficacy of pulmonary vein ablation was unknown then [in 2000] and it is unknown now... it is by far the most dangerous procedure ever performed in an electrophysiology lab."

It seemed extraordinary to no one in the room that a doctor was telling the Food and Drug Administration, an agency designed to safeguard the public, that he has been performing—and continues to perform—a procedure which he considers to be dangerous and unproven.

Calkins told the panel that cardiologists needed the REVELATION system so they'd have a procedure to perform while trying to figure out if pulmonary vein isolation was worth the risks—risks that Hugh Calkins was willing to take with other people's lives.

"What's nice about the REVELATION procedure," he said, "is that it's not a moving target. Here's three lesions which can be understood and are reproducible. It's clear how to deliver them. Where it fits in for a center like mine where we can do whatever we please, we'll tell the patients that they have an option. If they want to go for the home run, the cure, and they're willing to accept a procedure with higher risks that's in evolution and so forth, we're happy to go ahead and do a pulmonary vein isolation." But using the REVELATION, he said, would be "a better way to be approaching atrial fibrillation rather than just doing a high risk procedure right from the outset," which was the way that he was doing it.

The procedure he performed on Pam, or rather the procedure he let a cardiologist-in-training perform on Pam, was especially risky to her because it was difficult and complex to the point of being a challenge for the most skilled and experienced practitioners in the world. It was a tough procedure for doctors to get the hang of, let alone master.

"Anyone who is doing pulmonary vein ablation realizes there is a learning curve and the learning curve is very rocky as you go up on it and the complications are like no other procedure that's ever been done in an EP lab," Hugh Calkins said.

Having explained to the FDA panel how he'd helped to create a need for the product, Calkins launched into a defense of the integrity of the REVELATION investigational study. He put his Johns Hopkins reputation on the line and announced that "This study was very well designed, very well carried out, shows very sound data and very excellent safety."

His colleagues sitting on the FDA's Circulatory System Devices Panel didn't see it that way.

Dr. Leslie Ewing, the panel's Medical Director, started things off with a revelation of his own. Information had been leaked to him concerning what would turn out to be a relatively minor transgression: The study had been rigged.

According to the rules of the clinical study, patients were not to be told how many incidents of Afib they would have to experience in order to participate. Calkins had just informed the panel that as per the rules, "the patients were not told they had to cross a certain bar to get in." The thinking was that Afibbers, being offered what they thought was a chance of being cured, might exaggerate their symptoms in order to be eligible for the investigation.

Then Dr. Ewing announced that, contrary to what Hugh Calkins had just told the panel, "It is the FDA's information that the patients were aware that a minimum number of episodes were required."

Calkins & Co. had just gotten caught trying to put one over on the FDA, and things went downhill from there.

The voting members of the FDA panel had already read all the materials from Cardima's Pre-Market Approval request. Nobody was buying it. For beginners, there was general skepticism over the effectiveness of the right-sided ablations for atrial fibrillation. Dr. Roosevelt Gilliam from Duke University wondered if Calkins himself did the procedure.

"This question may not be playing fair but I do need to ask it," Gilliam said. "When you do your pulmonary vein ablations now, do you routinely do right-sided lines as this system would dictate?"

Calkins replied that he did not. "I think very few people are doing it. They aren't working on the right side routinely..." Everyone had moved on to the pulmonary veins.

Dr. Ewing proceeded to read a laundry list of Hugh Calkins's sins against science:

The primary investigators contaminated the data. In a clinical trial to determine the safety and effectiveness of Cardima's catheter system, Calkins told doctors that all they had to do was try using the Cardima catheter first, and then they were free to use whatever type of catheter they were most comfortable with. Which was a bad enough breach of the study protocol, but there was more: Dr. Christopher White, head of cardiology at Ochsner Heart and Vascular Institute in New Orleans, pointed out to Calkins that "You have a whole bunch of patients in here who weren't tried with your catheter at all."

Thus Calkins was proposing that the FDA approve an investigational device based partly on results achieved with a different piece of equipment. Further, the study data was collected and organized in such a haphazard way that there was no way to even know whether the patients had actually received any ablation treatment at all.

There was "a lack of rigor and discipline and investigators did not play by the rules." Calkins's presentation did not even rise to the level of a true clinical trial; the way it was set up and run, it was merely an observational exercise.

To sum up, Dr. Ewing said that because there was no way to determine the risk-benefit profile of the REVELATION system, the panel had determined that "from the clinical and statistical perspective, it is not clear if data can support any conclusion about the safety and effectiveness of the system."

The study was a complete bust, rejected outright due to incompetence and fraud, with each panel member in turn heaping scorn upon the effort.

Sharon-Lise T. Normand is a professor at Harvard Medical School who holds a doctorate in biostatistics from Toronto University. Zeroing in on the data, and the conspicuous lack thereof, she kindly affected a hint of dumb blonde. "I just look at the numbers and I keep getting different results," she said to Dr. Ewing. "Can you just go over it one more time?"

Dr. Ewing did his best, but Cardima's REVELATION study was such a Rubik's Cube that even a world-class statistician piled high and deep couldn't figure it out. "I just want to get a sense of why we're missing some data for the primary endpoint," Dr. Normand said.

"I know maybe the sponsor can tell me. Is it 87? Is it 83? Is it 81 and whether or not the 20 or 22, depending on how you count people?" she asked Calkins, and "Statistically you need to adjust for the fact that you have multiple centers. Didn't you adjust?" Calkins said no, he hadn't, adding, "I'm not a statistician," which was becoming more and more apparent.

As a matter of fact, for a Harvard trained research scientist, Professor Calkins appears to have a somewhat breezy attitude toward statistics. At a breakfast symposium hosted by Cardima in 2001, he explained how he crunched the numbers from Phase II of the REVELATION trial. "The results of the first 48 patients can be interpreted based on what type of person you are—an optimist or a pessimist," he said. "If you're a pessimist, you'd probably say, '47 out of 48 patients had atrial fibrillation again, so it doesn't work...'"

Dr. White was blunt about the sad excuse for science that Hugh Calkins had wrought. "My problem is that if you're sloppy enough to do the protocol this way then I think that runs through the whole study. That contaminates the study. You wrote the protocol and then you didn't stick to it. I don't like that. I don't quite understand the freedom of your investigators to deviate from the protocol. What was going on in their minds?" White said.

He added that "These would be protocol deviations that would come up as red flags right off the bat. I don't know why the waters were allowed to get so muddy."

Dr. David Schwartzman, a New Yorker, knew medicine from learning in the trenches at NYU and was not impressed by Ivy Leaguers. "I'm concerned that we're approving a protocol or a technology and technique that is going to end up being a waste of the physician and patient's time and money. My own personal experience with right atrial linear ablation is that only 10 percent of these patients remained without another procedure. So at the end of the day the long term benefit is hard to find," he said.

Schwartzman, in addition to believing that Calkins's theory was a waste of time and money, could see what was coming down the road if the scheme were approved. It seems that certain doctors— who shall remain nameless—were prone to get carried away with the technology at the expense of their patients. "I have concern regarding the safety of this technology and its inevitable use in the left atrium as soon as it gets into the hands of those of us who have our own visions about this technology," he said. "We get away with a tremendous amount in the heart as it is …" He spoke of "our arrogance about pulmonary veins and left atrial ablation"—a pointed reference to how far ahead of himself Hugh Calkins had gotten.

Unlike the rest of the panel, Dr. Schwartzman had little to say about how the study data was collected and organized. "I respect the statistical mischief here," he said. In other words, we all know what goes on, but Hugh Calkins, you have gone beyond decent.

Dr. Cynthia Tracy of Washington University Hospital thought the entire project was garbage.

"This study has many serious flaws," she said. "I don't think there's anything salvageable."

One of the flaws she cited was the deliberate under reporting of adverse events along with the overstatement of the success rate. "It appears that the sponsor is using a narrow interpretation of the standard definition of adverse events," she said, noting that had the rules been followed, the rate of adverse events would be 19% instead of 4%.

The success rate would have been 20%, not the 85% that Hugh Calkins claimed.

How important is it for doctors to be careful with study data? Dr. Roderick Tung, a cardiologist at UCLA's David Geffen School of Medicine thinks it is very important.

> "With modern medicine, less emphasis has been placed on the physician-patient dialogue where concerns and expectations are freely exchanged. Physicians should understand that choosing longevity with potential tradeoffs in device-related complications and quality of life is a personal decision that must be individually tailored to patient preference.

> "The process of obtaining informed consent from patients mandates and pre-supposes that physicians, first, are fully informed of the risks and benefits of the therapy that they are offering. It is ethically imperative that we are honest with the data, so that we can be honest with our patients."

Ethical imperatives took a back seat to expediency in the REVELATION study and in the end the FDA panel saw this effort for what it was, more PR than science.

"The spin you put on it I understand, and I'd love to believe you," said Dr. Waldo to Hugh Calkins.

Dr. Waldo could not believe the spin because he was a doctor and he knew better. But what if you were a trusting patient who fit the profile of a candidate for an experimental technique?

I had an ablation over 3 months ago and have had a cough from the time I got out of surgery until now. I have pericarditis without effusion and have to sleep propped up. They said that the machine blew a fuse when they were working on me and they had to wait 25 minutes until the janitor could replace it. My concerns are that they would not have any imaging system after the blown fuse, and could not see where the catheter was.

I think the catheter may take a while to cool, so I'm worried that it might have burned something it shouldn't have. My heart rate jumped 20 to 25 bpm (to 100) after the procedure and it was unsuccessful. I still get Afib up to 180 bpm.

Chapter 26

Personal and Confidential

HUGH CALKINS WAS the lead author, but Dr. Ron Berger received author credit for the journal article about Pam's complication, as did Richard Wu and Jeffrey Brinker. Quite an impressive byline, it represents more than $1 million worth of the finest education that money can buy—and they are all excellent dancers. The authors refer to the patient as *our* patient and Ron Berger is listed in the medical report as having actually participated in the procedure. So I was quite surprised by the reply from Ron Berger in 2005 concerning my request for his records of Pam's case.

"I have never been involved in your wife's care in any way," he wrote back.

It was four years after the fact and by then I was tired of being taken for a fool. I was pretty sure that tampering with the medical record and academic fraud would be frowned upon at JHU, so I wrote to the provost.

I was going to get Calkins and Berger into hot water because of what they did.

Stephen Knapp, (Yale, *Lux et Veritas*) who is now president at George Washington University, was then provost at Hopkins, the top enforcer of academic integrity. He responded:

PERSONAL AND CONFIDENTIAL
Office of the Provost
June 23, 2006
Dear Mr. Walter:

I am writing in response to your e-mail message to me dated July 16, 2005 regarding Dr. Ron Berger's role in the medical care of your wife.

The School of Medicine conducted a review of Dr. Berger's role in the medical care of your wife during her admission to the Johns Hopkins Hospital in March 2002 and his role as an author of the case report describing the complication that occurred during her surgery. The School's review concluded that Dr. Berger had no involvement in the medical care of your wife during her 2002 admission to Johns Hopkins.

You correctly point out that he is listed in the medical record as an "assistant" in the ablation procedure. We have determined that the listing was an error and it will be corrected.

The reviewers learned that during your wife's ablation procedure, the attending physicians informally consulted Dr. Berger concerning the complication that arose. Dr. Berger made no recommendations to the plan of care. Furthermore, because he was not involved in the ablation procedure, he did not compare the medical record and the case report, and was not responsible for any patient-related medical information in the case report.

Sincerely,
Steven Knapp, Ph.D.

It would appear from Provost Knapp's letter that when things got ugly down in the EP Lab, somebody called Ron Berger and said "You've gotta come down here and see this!" or something to that effect. So he was alerted to the botched ablation in progress in Room One of the EP Lab, but he "made no recommendations to the plan of care... was not involved in the ablation procedure... did not compare the medical record and the case report... and was not responsible for any patient-related medical information in the case report."

That's what passes for authorship in academic medicine.

But, as it turns out, the Provost was wrong. Ron Berger did take his turn attempting to undo the Gordian knot, so maybe he does rate an official assist in the ghost-ridden world of medical journals.

In addition to being confused as to who was actually in the room at the time, Calkins had trouble recalling how many sites were ablated inside Pam's heart. After Jeff Brinker unceremoniously liberated the catheter from Pam's mitral valve, and it was clear that a full-blown fiasco was in progress in his EP Lab, Doc Calkins must have decided it was time to make himself scarce, go talk to family members or make some phone calls, because apparently he left Pam in acute congestive heart failure with his understudies for a while, and it looks like some enterprising young Fellow or Resident or Intern—could have been anybody—showed some initiative and took the liberty to go ahead and ablate another site (do another burn) while the boss was away.

Because, while Calkins told me he only got two sites done, the medical record shows that three sites inside Pam's heart were ablated that day. He didn't know about the third one.

When you look at his notes of the procedure, it was clear that he had written up his report with the two sites ablated and then the entanglement of the mitral valve, and then he signed it.

Sometime later he wrote under his signature: "Addendum: We proceeded to isolate the RSPV (Right Superior Pulmonary Vein) successfully."

"The attending performed the procedure," says Calkins for the record. And he writes that as soon as the assembled senior cardiology staff saw the shredded particles of flesh clinging to the tip of the catheter pulled from Pam's heart, they immediately called the surgeons and rushed to prep her for surgery. In reality, Calkins had wandered away from a patient who was critically injured—and the ablation procedure was then continued without his knowledge on a patient who had just suffered a life-threatening trauma and who was dying by the minute.

But, initially, as far as Calkins knew, two sites were ablated and that's what he told everyone. That's what he told me. That's what he told Pam's daughter. Given the cascading calamities in progress, the beleaguered Calkins probably felt he had to stick with that story and hope that we'd never find out.

How many screw-ups can a doctor admit to in one day?

Chapter 27

Respiratory Compromise

"*ICU Subsequent Care Note:* Delirium; pt remains very agitated on fentanyl and received dose of haldol this AM. Will again attempt to decrease fentanyl but we have not had any success. Once it is decreased she becomes agitated and has respiratory compromise. We will continue to attempt to wean fentanyl so that we may assess her for extubation. Neuro consult obtained."

EXCEPT FOR THE LIGHTING, it was as bleak inside the 5th Floor ICU as it was out on the rain-swept streets of Baltimore. Fluorescent white shown upon the linens of the dying and the recovering alike—and upon Pam, who was stuck somewhere in between, in a world of bruises and stitches and blood and gauze. For all the chirping electronics and humming machines and dripping drips, she wouldn't wake up. She was spiking fevers of unknown origin. Grim fluids oozed through a tube that had been inserted between her ribs.

All the while, her eyes were only halfway shut and she stared vacantly into the exam light that seemed to be always hovering overhead at full intensity. I told the nurses more than a few times that her eyes needed some drops or lubrication—or something. Doctors were in a Catch-22 trying to wean Pam off the ventilator. When they reduced the sedatives so she could start breathing on her own, she began to gag on the tube that was down her throat, which made it impossible for them to get it out.

"ETT repositioned to right side of mouth by RT.
Pt more awake and restless, coughing and gagging."

I can see it as if it were happening right now, right in front of me. Gagging on the ventilator tube lodged in her throat, choking and gagging, wrists tied to the bed rails and she pulling against them, pulling herself up from the bed, heaving forward, straining, neck muscles taught, breastbone split, bones scraping, choking, the pressure popping her eyes open, red veined and raw, hot tears, and the fierce frantic struggle for air, for breath, for life itself.

Then sedation and then calm for a while.

Now I understood what she had sensed after the botched ablation, in the foreboding over open-heart surgery—that sooner or later they will kill her. She would never get out alive and I'd been wrong to reassure her, I'd been wrong to believe in this place, wrong to bring her here.

Chapter 28

A Drink of Water

MEANWHILE, down in Pediatrics, they were preparing the groundwork for the launch of the Josie King Patient Safety Program. Josie King was 18 months old when she was taken to Hopkins after being scalded in a bathtub accident in February 2001, a year before Pam's encounter with the culture of safety.

"She healed well and within weeks was scheduled for release," Josie's mother, Sorrel King, writes on the Josie King Foundation website.

But something was wrong. Josie seemed to be very thirsty all the time, eagerly seeking moisture from any available source. Sorrell King knew her daughter was desperately thirsty, and she wanted to give her water, but was told she couldn't. She deferred to the experts.

The little girl died from dehydration.

The Summer, 2004 online issue of *Hopkins Medicine* features a story called *A Remedy of Errors*, an audacious work of public relations, which I predict one day will make it to the University of Spin as a textbook example of how to write when you've been handed a lemon of a story:

> *"Out of a deadly medical mistake at Hopkins Hospital sprang a patient safety effort that has united a bereaved parent with malpractice lawyers, physicians and nurses."*

The story starts out with a visit to the home of Josie's parents by the Director of the Johns Hopkins Children's Center, Dr. George Dover: "What could he possibly say to this man and woman whose 18-month-old daughter had died at Hopkins just days earlier, not of some rare, incurable disease but of thirst?"

"We knew what had happened," says Sorrell King. "We wanted someone to tell us why—why didn't they listen to us when we said something was wrong with Josie, why didn't they give her something to drink? We were involved with our lawyer then. We were going for it. If George had said, 'We're not sure what happened,' we would have thrown him out."

George knew exactly what to say.

The Kings had hired Paul D. Bekman to represent them. Hopkins was faced with the nightmare prospect of a junkyard dog like Bekman holding the personal injury lawyer's straight flush: a slam dunk case involving the death of a child—a child of the upper middle class. Hopkins definitely wanted to stop the King family from "going for it."

"My husband, our lawyer and George were holding me back from going to the newspapers," says Sorrell. So when Doc Dover visited the King family at their home on that "windy March Sunday," he was all contrition. Hopkins was quick to settle with the Kings for an undisclosed sum and they agreed to help set up the Josie King Foundation. They did not do these things because it was the right thing to do. They did them because there was nothing else they could do. There was no blaming the victim in this case. There were no consent forms or technicalities to hide behind. They had killed a pretty little girl.

As president of The Johns Hopkins Hospital back in 1999, Ron Peterson was a hard charging executive with an eye for innovation —and he had a special interest in patient safety because his father died because of a medical mistake. One day he read a report from the Institute of Medicine which detailed the sad state of patient safety in America. One hundred thousand people a year died from medical mistakes and some of those tragic deaths might have been prevented.

According to the Baltimore Sun, Ron Peterson "understood the report's call to action." What was needed was a plan, a grand plan to make patient safety not merely a top priority at the Hopkins— but *The Number One Priority.*

Two years later, as Josie King lay dying for want of a drink of water, Peterson and other Hopkins visionaries were "still hammering out their plans" for patient safety.

If patient safety wasn't *The Number One Priority* at Johns Hopkins Medicine, what was?

It was and is the same number one priority of any business: to make money. And the business model is this: Aggressively projecting and protecting the image of being the best hospital in America, and using that reputation to attract patients, who are treated by underpaid and overworked students of medicine. The big names lure them in and the residents and interns, who covet the Hopkins name for their resumes, do the work for dirt metered out by corporate medicine.

The Baltimore Sun ran a feature story about the Josie King tragedy. Hopkins management responded with righteous outrage at their own failings, and a declaration of resolve to do better.

"Josie died of a Third World disease—dehydration—in the best hospital in the world," said Dr. Peter J. Pronovost, a Hopkins physician and patient safety expert, whose father had been the victim of a medical mistake.

"How could that possibly happen? The answer is, we've created a system that's allowed it to happen."

Proclamations were issued from on High:

"I want everybody in the hospital empowered to be able to pull a cord and stop the assembly line when they see something unsafe," said Dr. William R. Brody, president of the Johns Hopkins University.

There were mea culpas and calls for accountability:

"This is my hospital. This happened on my watch," said Dr. George Dover. "This is my responsibility. I'll get to the bottom of it." Dover said that what had happened to Josie was a sentinel event – an unexpected occurrence resulting in serious injury or death. He said a committee would be formed to review what had happened and recommend ways to correct any problems.

And, to demonstrate sincerity and a willingness to go the extra mile, Dr. Dover promised that the hospital would try not to cover anything up.

"By June 2001, four months after Josie died, Hopkins had finished its review and told Sorrel and Tony what they had known all along: Josie's death had resulted from a total breakdown of the system," the Sun reported.

"Three weeks into her recovery, the child had suffered devastating brain damage after her heart stopped because of severe dehydration. The medical staff hadn't responded appropriately to the warning signs—her precipitous weight loss, severe diarrhea, intense thirst and lethargy."

Dr. Dover may have taken full responsibility for the senseless death of Josie King, but when the internal investigation finally got to the bottom of it all, they found that a temp nurse should take the fall: "the committee concluded that the temporary agency nurse tending to Josie the day her heart stopped should have been more aggressive in alerting physicians to the child's symptoms."

Richard P. Kidwell, Hopkins' managing attorney for claims and litigation, said, "The information was there, but no one really put it all together."

Kidwell later revealed that the committee's investigation had determined that the desperately desiccated Josie King should have been given a drink of water.

However, as the Baltimore Sun said, out of tragedy sprang a passion for safety, and the desire for Johns Hopkins to become the world leader in patient safety. The Josie King Foundation would light the way of safe passage for all the sick and injured in the dicey environs of John Hopkins Medicine.

Chapter 29

Two Months Later

Johns Hopkins Admits Fault in Fatal Experiment

ELLEN ROCHE was a healthy 24-year-old lab technician. In June of 2001, she pulled a flyer off a bulletin board and went to make a few extra bucks by participating in a study. It was an 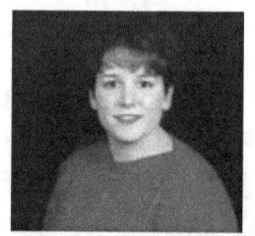 asthma study, and the participants were left to the assumption that the researchers wanted to test the effectiveness of a new medicine.

So, for $365, Ellen Roche inhaled the gas, and then, basically, her lungs shriveled up. She spent several weeks in the ICU before her parents removed life support. Perhaps if hexamethonium had been listed on the consent form as the drug that she would be inhaling, lab tech Roche might have looked it up on Google, where several sites would have told her that she was in danger.

Hexamethonium was known to cause lung damage; indeed, that was the reason they were giving it to people, and they were giving it in amounts that some doctors characterized as 'extraordinarily large'—amounts that the FDA would certainly not have approved had they been asked.

The FDA cited lack of informed consent as one of the many study violations.

"Failure to obtain effective informed consents from subjects, in that the sponsor/clinical investigator failed to disclose that inhalation administration of hexamethonium was an experimental use of the drug." Participants were told that the main risk was a temporary drop in blood pressure. That's what it said on the consent form.

University of Iowa Law Professor Nicholas Johnson maintains that Ellen Roche and the other study subjects were unaware of the full extent of the risks to which they were being subjected—such as death from the total destruction of their lungs.

The 'medication' that they were administered was in fact a lung irritant, a chemical that lost FDA approval for its original intended purpose in 1972. It was not approved by the FDA for this study. It was being used experimentally, and at no time in its history had it ever been approved in an inhaled form. Johnson says that Hopkins researchers deliberately used a chemical they knew would worsen the subjects' lung condition, which in fact was the purpose of the study: "To find out how the tubes that carry air into the lungs can stay open even when we breathe irritating chemicals."

Johns Hopkins researchers wanted to study the ways in which people with asthma respond to substances that constricted their airways.

They were deliberately harming people, deliberately causing asthma attacks in healthy subjects—and they did it all with the full permission of management. It was a big scandal and made the papers for a couple of months. The Office of Human Research Protections suspended almost all medical research involving human subjects at Johns Hopkins. The FDA and the Department of Health and Human Services also investigated the case and found that a Hopkins ethics committee and the Hopkins Institutional Review Board had approved the study.

Management was caught flat-footed in the press, but quickly pulled together its damage control act. The Baltimore Sun reported that "Hopkins leaders initially chose to reveal little, at the risk of appearing to have something to hide."

Then they settled on a strategy of mea culpas and promises of reform, including stirring words from the CEO. "Her loss can hold meaning for the whole Hopkins family if it reminds us of our obligation to protect the lives of those who seek our help," said Ed Miller.

Ed Miller said that Ellen Roche had not necessarily died in vain; her death could serve to remind Johns Hopkins Medicine that it has an obligation to safeguard its patients. A much needed reminder for Johns Hopkins, but it appears not to have had any such effect.

The same month that Ellen Roche died, Hopkins got a letter from the FDA that described the shoddy doings at their Breast Imaging Center as "serious underlying problems that could compromise the quality of mammography performed at your facility, and represent a violation of the law."

In August 2001, the New York Times ran this story by Tamar Lewin:

U.S. Investigating Johns Hopkins Study of Lead Paint Hazard

BALTIMORE - Amid growing concern about the safety of medical research involving humans, the Department of Health and Human Services opened an investigation on Wednesday into a lead-paint study in Baltimore overseen by Johns Hopkins University.

The study was criticized last week in a decision by the Maryland Court of Appeals, which likened it to the infamous Tuskegee syphilis study decades ago. 'It can be argued that the researchers intended that the children be the canaries in the mines but never clearly told the parents," Judge Dale R. Cathell said in a scathing decision that compared the Baltimore study to Nazi medical experiments and the study in Tuskegee, Ala., that withheld treatment from black men with syphilis..

Suzanne Shapiro, the lawyer for Catina Higgins, one of the mothers who filed suit, said that in May, 1994... when Ms. Higgins and her 4-year-old son, Myron, moved into a rented house at 1906 East Federal Street, the lead in Myron's blood was at a safe level and his mother knew nothing about the study.

"After she moved in, Kennedy Krieger enrolled her in the study, and she signed the informed consent, but no one ever told her, 'There's lead in this house, and it can cause brain damage," said Ms. Shapiro. Ms. Shapiro said that a month later Myron's blood contained excessive lead, and that he had since had neurological problems.

The study which the Maryland Court of Appeals likened to Nazi medical experiments and the Tuskegee syphilis atrocity was approved by the Johns Hopkins Internal Review Board.

Manuel Roig-Franzia reported in the Washington Post that, despite the uproar, two other lead paint studies continued at the institute. In one, half of the participants—children ages one to eight—received a drug known to reduce elevated levels of lead in the blood, while the other half receive a placebo.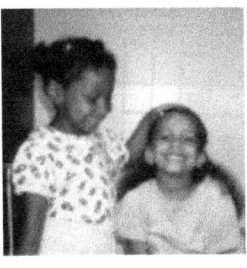

The March, 2000, issue of the New England Journal of Medicine reported on another study that was even more similar to Tuskegee. In a Hopkins research effort in Uganda, people were intentionally exposed to AIDS without their knowledge. They monitored 415 couples of which only one partner was infected with HIV. The researchers did not inform the AIDS-free partners.

They wanted to see what would happen, which was that two and a half years later, 90 of the formerly healthy spouses had become infected.

From the November, 2001 *British Medical Journal*:

Johns Hopkins Admits Scientist
used Indian Patients as Guinea Pigs

"The university announced last week that it had initiated sanctions against the scientist for participating in clinical trials that did not meet the university's standards for human research. The scientist had provided the drug to doctors at the Regional Cancer Centre in India's southern state of Kerala. The doctors injected a drug into 26 patients with oral cancer between November 1999 and April 2000. The university declined to name the scientist ..."

Management, of course, was shocked to discover that one of their researchers was playing fast and loose with the rules—even if it was in India. The researcher was sanctioned, banned, exiled. Further, it was announced that the practice of using patients as guinea pigs would no longer be tolerated at Johns Hopkins.

Chapter 30

The Gravy Train

*"Biotech Industry, Universities Oppose State Oversight
of Medical Research"* — Baltimore Sun

THE PRACTICE of using people as guinea pigs may have been publicly renounced, but Hopkins was not about to abandon the business model.

The death of Ellen Roche caught the attention of legislators in Annapolis, who had until now been happy to leave regulation of Nazi medical experiments and Tuskegee syphilis studies to the Feds. The recent ghoulish headlines out of Baltimore, however, had incited state lawmakers to action. The Baltimore Sun's Tom Pelton wrote about voluntary oversight, which meant there was virtually no regulation of medical experiments being conducted on human beings. Hopkins and other research hospitals were not required to report injuries or deaths of research subjects.

"It's an honor system," said Arthur Caplan, director of the University of Pennsylvania's Bioethics Program. "Many adverse events do not get reported because doctors and researchers don't like to think about themselves causing harm. So if there's something else to blame it on, like an illness, they will." At the Sun, Pelton asked for "adverse event" figures from the review boards of the University of Maryland and Johns Hopkins. UM released the numbers from their medical school. Of the approximately 1,000 experiments conducted the previous year, there were 880 reports of "serious adverse events" suffered by volunteers.

Johns Hopkins refused to release any figures.

A state legislator responded by introducing a bill that would shed some light on the whole human research situation, which alarmed the people who ran the show in Baltimore, who feared that transparency and rules to protect patients would derail the Federal Research Gravy Train—an express with daily nonstops from the U.S. Treasury to Johns Hopkins Inc.

Physics Today reported in 2009 that Johns Hopkins University was the biggest recipient of US R&D funds for the 30th year in a row, pulling in more than $3 billion from federal agencies like the National Institutes of Health and the Department of Defense, as well as funding from foundations and industry.

So, ten days before Pam was wheeled into Room One of the Hopkins EP Lab under false pretenses, the leaders of the state's biotech and medical research industry descended upon the State Capitol in Annapolis to educate lawmakers on the issues of informed consent and patient safety. The message to the legislature was that despite recent unpleasantness, the current hodgepodge of federal regulation was working fine. Why mess with a good thing?

It was a good thing for Hopkins, Inc. because federal law did not cover most of what they did up there.

There were many supporters of the state bill. It had 16 co-sponsors, as well as the support of the state attorney general's office and two patient safety organizations.

Hopkins vice president Joanne Pollak told the Baltimore Sun that her institution certainly supported the *general concept* of meaningful oversight. "We support anything that will build the trust of people in participating in the good research that is going on at Hopkins and other institutions in the state," she said. However, in her humble opinion, the state bill needed some work.

What these well-intended reformers didn't understand, Pollack explained, was that there was money at stake. A lot of money. She said that the huge flow of federal research dollars into the area would evaporate overnight if the state law got passed as written. She could fix that with an amendment that would make the new state laws compatible with existing federal laws. As a matter of fact, Hopkins had more (and better) lawyers than the legislature, and so they just went ahead and wrote up a new version of the bill, which would be compatible with federal law.

The Hopkins bill was more than compatible with Federal law. It was identical.

"This will ensure that research institutions and researchers in Maryland are not disadvantaged when competing for federally funded and other sponsored research," Pollack said.

A little more back and forth with some key players out in the hallway, and then a done deal, problem solved. HB 917 passed the Maryland House of Delegates by a vote of 135 to 1 on March 25th, 2002, the date of Pam's admission to Johns Hopkins hospital—and the date she was declared to be disabled by the United States Social Security Administration.

Before the final vote, one lawmaker actually read the final draft. And he saw that a change had been made that wasn't part of the deal. It was an amendment that gutted the legislature's sunshine provision of the law, which allowed for public access to safety records.

Oops, said Pollak, how did that get in there?

The February 2002 issue of JHU Magazine carried a Special Report headlined *Trials & Tribulations*, about what a rough time the institution had been having lately.

"Last summer's painful events have forced the university to confront tough questions about its program for ensuring patient safety in clinical research trials. The question now is, where does Johns Hopkins go from here?"

They didn't go anywhere. Publishing what they considered to be a self-flagellating magazine article appeared to be the extent of actions they'd take in response to the exposure of their cavalier attitude toward patient safety.

"Roche's death, the first death ever of a healthy volunteer at Johns Hopkins, stunned Hopkins researchers. They were stunned again on July 19 when the U.S. Office for Human Research Protections (OHRP) suspended all federally funded research involving human subjects at nearly all Hopkins divisions."

The defensive tone of the article tells you all you need to know about the future of journalism when taught at a university steeped in corporate culture:

The shutdown halted some 2,400 protocols. The initial response from the university was anger: A media release on the day of the suspension called OHRP's action 'unwarranted, unnecessary, paralyzing, and precipitous,' and you can still find researchers who--not for attribution-- use the words 'excessive' and 'disproportionate' and 'bordering on unethical.' Hopkins nonetheless accepted responsibility...

The findings from both committees forced Johns Hopkins to confront inadequacies in its protection of human research subjects. And Hopkins administrators and faculty began a long, painful process of institutional soul-searching...

At a town meeting last July, Edward Miller, chief executive officer of Johns Hopkins Medicine, made it clear that he believed Hopkins had to do more than just tweak its review process. 'There has got to be a cultural change here,' Miller said. Chief executive officers do not just toss around the phrase 'cultural change. Miller challenged his colleagues to examine their fundamental approach to research on human volunteers.

He exhorted them to go well beyond whatever the government required, to establish a new benchmark for human research subject protection. 'We're going to have to raise the bar higher,' Miller said. 'There can't be any slippage. None.'

This was the issue of JHU Magazine that was scattered on coffee tables throughout the hospital and university on the day that Pam was wheeled into Room 101 for her procedure. Apparently some chief executives *do* just toss around the phrase "cultural change."

In 2003, Hopkins responded to a letter from the Office of Human Research Protection concerning a study underway involving the integrity of silicone breast implants: "JHU concedes that the above-referenced human subjects research was conducted without appropriate IRB review and approval and without informed consent."

And they got another warning from the FDA that year:

"A recent letter from the Food and Drug Administration to Johns Hopkins University in Baltimore contains what may prove to be the start of agency efforts to bring unregulated human experimentation under federal oversight, according to BNA interviews with key FDA personnel," wrote reporter M. Alexander Otto for *BNA's Medical Research Law & Policy Report.*

Chapter 31

Fine Wood Furniture

DAY AFTER DAY AFTER DAY Pam lay in a coma.

Hugh Calkins would occasionally make an appearance when a new family member arrived. When Pam's sister flew in from Seattle, he told her the same story that he'd told the rest of us: that he'd turned away momentarily during the procedure and the catheter got caught in her mitral valve muscles.

Sorry, he says, again and again, but now it was starting to have a ring of *tough luck* to it. Sorry. Oops. Oh, well. And as the days wore on, we began to see less and less of Hugh Calkins.

I had assumed that once the *complication* had occurred, Pam would be receiving extra-special attention. I had a rube's fantasies about her being taken care of in the Marburg Pavilion, the section of the hospital behind velvet ropes which offers luxurious care to the fabulously wealthy at a comfortable remove from the great unwashed:

"The Marburg Pavilion offers deluxe accommodations for a limited number of adult patients who desire not only the finest medical care, but also the utmost in comfort and privacy. Located within the historic Marburg Building of The Johns Hopkins Hospital, the Pavilion is more reminiscent of a five-star luxury hotel than a hospital.

"These tastefully decorated private rooms and suites feature fine wood furniture, private baths, entertainment centers, and an array of special amenities. Yet each room is fully equipped to deliver the most advanced medical care. For beneath its paneling and designer fabrics, the Marburg Pavilion is, above all, a modern, technically sophisticated, hospital facility. Although connected to the main hospital building, public access to the Pavilion floor is limited. This helps to create a quiet, less stressful environment, conducive to your recuperation.

"What's more, a dedicated, multifunctional team — from nurses to guest services staff — is assigned to each patient. So you will always find a familiar face to assist you. But more importantly, you can be confident that every team member understands your particular medical needs and personal requirements, including your business needs."

I thought maybe being dangled over the precipice of death would qualify you for "an array of special amenities," or at least land you in a "quiet, less stressful environment." The Pavilion, however, was off limits to those who had to worry about deductibles: "Rooms in the Marburg Pavilion are available at an additional charge."

So, instead of having "a dedicated, multifunctional team—from nurses to guest services staff" assigned to her, Pam's odds of survival depended on an overburdened and sleep-deprived Resident who was working close to 100 hours a week—and he was certainly not a familiar face to any of us.

One morning I walked into the ICU and found that Pam was lying on her side and curling up into what looked like a fetal position, her knees beginning to draw up, her hands heading toward communion under her chin. I asked a nurse to take a look at her.

"Don't worry," she told me.

But I knew better. I'd seen it before. This is a person curling up to die, like autumn's last dead leaf, and we, as a family, demanded to see the doc in charge.

But he was a hard man to get a hold of, and an article in The American Medical News explains why:

Johns Hopkins Penalized for Resident Hour Violations

"The Accreditation Council for Graduate Medical Education has disciplined its first resident program for work-hour violations since new rules went into effect for all programs July 1. Johns Hopkins Hospital's internal medicine program was cited for exceeding the 80-hour work week and requiring call more than every third night in the intensive care, counter to ACGME work hour standards."

The council's rebuke had no impact. Johns Hopkins Magazine dutifully reported that "Nine days into the new enforcement period, a new Hopkins intern sent an e-mail to ACGME officials stating that some Internal Medicine residents were working more than 100 hours per week."

I tracked our elusive resident doctor for days, finally pinning him down at a nurse's station. The man was obviously exhausted, but so was I, and I pressed him about why no one was doing anything about Pam's obvious trajectory toward her grave. His exasperation showing, he told me more or less that he was a very busy guy, with lots of patients—and they all had families who wanted answers—and he had a family of his own to worry about.

Chapter 32

I'll wait

I DON'T REMEMBER the name of the Chief of Cardiac Surgery, but I do know he had a really big office, a really nice office. The double doors were always wide open, indicating an admirable management philosophy.

From my perch at the edge of the sofa in the reception area, I spent a lot of time examining the details of the room, which seemed to exude a warm glow and was very nicely trimmed out. From my angle, I could see the books on the coffee table and the crossed legs of supplicants and applicants. I could hear the cordial tone of the conversations in which transactions were made and business was conducted. All very genteel up here, and civilized, above all the messy flesh asunder on the floors below.

On the second day of my vigil, the Chief reconsidered his open door policy.

Now it was just the secretary and I in the outer office. I smiled at the visitors as the doors opened for them, and closed. I smiled as they came and went. I could sense the secretary's frequent and furtive glances at me. Thank you, I'll wait, I'd said, and I'd meant it.

At some point she picked up the phone and said yes and then a few seconds later the door opened. The doc stood on the threshold and smiled. I was ushered in. I was in a big chair, looking across a big desk at the silver haired Chief, who was calm, confident and pleasant. His eyes were exceptionally clear, the color of Ice Blue Aqua Velva.

"What can I do for you?"

I was going to get tough with him. I was going to tell him that if my wife died it wouldn't be good for anybody, and that he'd better get down there and fix this problem.

I was going to tell him that I used to make my living putting headlines in the newspapers and that I was good at it. People would know what went on here.

But the only thing I wound up telling him was that I was afraid that my wife was going to die.

And the truth is that I was more than afraid. I was starting to really believe it.

The Chief told me that he would find out what was happening and that I should come back to see him first thing in the morning.

I could have watched the sunrise the next morning, but there was rain. I was in the hall outside his office watching raindrops weave their way down tall plate glass windows when the Chief walked up to me. I hadn't seen him coming. He put his hand on my shoulder and smiled.

"Don't worry," he said. "Your wife's not going to die."

A nurse later told me that she'd been working there for four years and this was the first time anybody had seen him down on the factory floor.

Chapter 33
Patient Combative

      "Many healthcare professionals believe that ICU psychosis and other changes in mental status are caused by factors inherent in the critical care environment, such as the constant noise, frequent interruptions, windowless rooms, overwhelming and unfamiliar technology, and the lack of orientation clues."

      — *Brenda Hixon-Vermillion, RN, BSN*

IT WAS AROUND 1 AM when the nurses called. I pulled on some jeans and a shirt and walked over to the hospital, more than a little nervous in the middle of the Baltimore night.

After three weeks, they'd been able to get the breathing tube out of her and she was slowly emerging from the coma. But the long stay in the ICU had taken its toll.

It seems that Pam had been making a ruckus. She was arguing with the nurse, demanding nickels and dimes so she could use the pay phone which she saw hanging from the IV pole next to the bed. "My husband told me I could call him anytime and he'd be right here. He said even if I was only scared I should call him! I want to talk to my husband!"

The nurse alternated between an irritated, patronizing tone and genuine kindness, repeatedly informing Pam that it was all in her head and that there was in fact no telephone there. Pam accused the nurse of conspiring to keep her from talking with her husband.

She had lost her mind, which is not uncommon in intensive care units.

"Most critical care nurses are familiar with the term ICU psychosis," writes Nurse Manager Brenda Hixon-Vermillion of the Ohio State University Medical Center's ICU. She defines it as "a disorder in which patients in an ICU or similar setting experience anxiety, have visual and/or auditory hallucinations, become paranoid, agitated, and potentially violent, and may become disoriented to time and place."

Patients who have extended stays in ICUs, which Hixon-Vermillion defines as anything longer than two or three weeks, are more prone to the development of serious psychological and cognitive problems. Most critical care nurses are familiar with the term ICU psychosis. Brown cites studies which show that approximately one in every three patients who spend more than five days in a critical care unit will experience some sort of psychotic reaction.

Pam came back to us in stages. Tubes and needles and clips and wires were removed in their turn, leaving behind scars, puncture wounds, bruises and adhesive stuck to raw skin. Loving hands did a lot to coax her back to the land of the living as her mother and her daughter and sisters bathed her and washed her hair and painted her toenails.

Grimy little lines and pills of gray adhesive were scrubbed from her skin with refreshingly coarse hospital washcloths soaked in a basin of warm water with a little hotel bar of Ivory soap. They bought her new pajamas.

They wanted to help make her feel like a human being again. When she was awake they talked to her constantly and little by little her mind and her personality began to return to her. When they washed her hair, they found that it had gotten badly matted in the back. Pam's bed had been raised so that she was more or less sitting up. Mother and daughter stood on either side of the bed, debating various methods of untangling the knot of hair on the back of her head, turning it this way and that as if examining a melon at the farmer's market. Pam opened her eyes and said, "For Pete's sake, just cut the thing off."

The psychosis slowly faded, but, because of the stroke, she had trouble with her short-term memory. Her eyes were raw looking. One morning a student group from the Wilmer Eye Clinic was making rounds.

The professor examined Pam's eyes as the trainees look on. "Yep," he said confidently, "Exposure Keratopathy. When the eyelids stay open, the eyes dry out. There will be permanent damage to the corneas." And, he told them, "You'll see a lot of this in the ICU." He wrote an order for eye drops and the group moved on.

The long siege of oppressive gloom in the ICU gave way to optimism once Pam was moved to a step-down unit.

From there she went to a private room, and assessments began. They did a series of tests on her to assess the damage from the stroke. A therapist laid out all the makings for a sandwich and asked her to build one. After a few tries, she wound up with a piece of bread between two slices of cheese that were still wrapped in plastic.

The right side of her lower right arm constantly burned and tingled from nerve damage in her elbow. During her delirious phase in the CCU, they tied her arms to the bed, leaving one elbow resting on the rail so long that her ulnar nerve was damaged, which feels like the white-hot electric buzz you get when you hit your funny bone—only it never stops.

The scar down the middle of her chest was about eight inches long, and would replace cleavage as the main attraction of any low cut blouse or V-neck. Her balance was off and she could not walk without help for a long time. The scratched corneas meant she would never drive a car at night again.

She is now obliged to manage the high wire balancing act of taking the blood thinner warfarin for the rest of her life. Warfarin is commonly used as rat poison.

We got her out of there on the day before her 50th birthday. Three and a half weeks after I'd taken Pam to Johns Hopkins Hospital, I pushed her wheel chair out the front door.

Dazed, battered and bruised, with fewer parts than she came in with and a bald patch on the back of her head, she blinked into the April sunshine and smiled.

Chapter 34

Not the Answer

DURING A DINNER symposium at the Westin Copley Place hotel in Boston in 2006, just before they brought out the crème brulée, Hugh Calkins began a frank, shoptalk presentation on the results of his investigative studies.

"So really where I became enamored with Afib ablation, with this pulmonary approach, was when the Lasso catheter was developed by the group in Bordeaux. And the idea was that you have a circular catheter in the pulmonary vein, you can then go and electrically isolate the vein, ablating outside the valve ring and basically achieve the same thing," Calkins said.

"Now, I learned a lot of things the hard way about the Lasso catheter. One way, you can lasso lots of things with it, including the mitral valve and if you happen to Lasso the mitral valve it's very hard to untangle the valve and when we tried to untangle it, we ended up ripping the valve and having to replace the valve, and so that was a memorable Lasso experience," he said.

In a room full of doctors, Calkins took a swipe at the legal profession's ignorance of anatomical matters. "Just keep in mind, and then of course they tell you, the lawyers tell you, well in the package instructions it says, you know, never place this near the mitral valve. Well if you know where the pulmonary veins are, they're very near the mitral valve, so it's very hard not to lasso the valve occasionally," he said. "So anyhow, I went ahead and started doing the procedure and the results that I saw in our first 75 patients..."

The results weren't pretty: a 52% success rate and complications galore: "When you think about complications, they were memorable, two strokes, three tamponades, the mitral valve lassoed, an occluded pulmonary vein, some vascular complications..." Calkins said.

The Lassoed mitral valve, of course, belonged to Pam. She and 74 other people underwent a technically challenging high-risk procedure performed by a trainee in order to determine whether a theory should be put into practice — and the answer was no.

The next group of 75 patients was treated with the circumferential method, and the results of that investigation were even worse, a 35% success rate and a 7% complication rate.

"One of the problems was pulmonary vein stenosis," Calkins said. "A typical case is someone who had pulmonary vein ablation shows up in the ER with three pulmonary veins completely blocked and the fourth one 90% blocked. The patient gets emergency heart surgery and dies. Another person gets an Afib ablation, you get a call, the patient has been diagnosed with lung cancer, well it wasn't lung cancer, it was an occluded pulmonary vein that appeared to be lung cancer, but the patient got a lung removed. There was this iatrogenic epidemic of pulmonary vein stenosis… So, a 52% success rate, 6% complication rate, four deaths, so on and so forth …"

So on and so forth. That's just how the EP cookie crumbles.

"When I talked to my colleagues, they said well this problem of collateral damage happens everywhere, and all of us have to think about collateral damage…" Calkins said. "I learned a lot of things the hard way… with persistent and permanent Afib, this procedure was really awful – at the end you had about a 20% success rate. So the segmental ablation strategy really was not very impressive."

He tossed in a telling comment about having to repeat the procedure if it didn't take the first time, when he would tell the patient they were in need of a *touch up*. Referring to success rates in the published studies, he says "If you have a catheter ablation and you're getting it done again three months later, either the billables are a little down or else the patient failed the first procedure."

Calkins laid out a situation assuming the latter.

"And so we said let's take a harsh look at our numbers and see how we really did, and it was somewhat appalling. I think our success rate was about 35% for twelve month single procedure success rate, with a 7% complication rate."

This was the study in which Calkins later said that the numbers were so bad that his partner Ron Berger told him not to publish it, saying "We'd never get anymore Afib patients." Calkins said what he did was to find a successful subset of patients for whom the procedure seemed to have some effect and lead the article with that.

"And so we found a silver lining. We identified a subset of patients with paroxysmal Afib that were young and had a small left atrium and had blue eyes and had a 70% success rate—but for the rest the success rate was much worse."

"So I didn't feel this was the answer," he said. "At least for the patients that I had to deal with, and deal with the aftermath."

Calkins told the symposium crowd that it all worked out OK for him; his team won a prize.

"So we sent the paper in to be published to the Heart Rhythm Journal and it got rejected, but I sent it in again and I said this is a really important piece of paper, but it got rejected again. So I sent it in to the Journal of Interventional EP and they took it and I sent it in to the Heart Rhythm meeting and I had sort of a mixed reaction and my fellow called all delighted and he said that 'I just heard that I just won the Eric Prystowsky Clinical Research Prize from the Heart Rhythm Society and I said well, my goodness, fantastic, so then I went to Eric and I said what is this prize, and apparently the prize is for the top scoring clinical abstract at the meeting submitted by a fellow – anonymously – so of all of the abstracts submitted, this 32% success rate abstract was number one, so there he was today at his presentation, big award and all the rest of it with these awful results."

Chapter 35

The Before and the Aftermath

SO HUGH CALKINS had to "deal with the aftermath," of having let trainees perform an unprecedentedly risky procedure. How he dealt with it, I don't know. But I'm pretty sure his life went on just like before.

The aftermath dealt to Pam, however, constituted a whole different life for her. There was her life before, in the car on the way up to Baltimore, generally healthy and financially secure, an RN running her own business, telling me a joke, happy as she'd ever been.

After was disability. After was pain and pills and medical bills, anxiety and stress, doubt and depression.

At first, I really believed that Johns Hopkins would do something about it. The doctor said that Pam got hurt because he had turned away from the procedure. He took his eye off the ball and now Pam was disabled and disfigured. It seemed pretty clear cut to me. But according to Hopkins it was a known risk of the procedure—simultaneously claiming that it wasn't their fault because it was an unknown, previously unreported complication.

And Pam had signed a broadly worded consent form.

Chapter 36
They Didn't Cut you did they?

MALPRACTICE LAWYER Paul Bekman has an office in downtown Baltimore with window walls overlooking center field at Camden Yards, where the Baltimore Orioles play.

The man is obviously wildly successful, and over the years has developed "a relationship with Johns Hopkins," which is how he put it to me. Bekman and Hopkins see each other as someone you can do business with.

For example, Baltimore Sun investigative reporter Fred Schulte wrote that "Lawyers who sue Maryland's elite hospitals for alleged medical mistakes often don't target the physicians involved, a practice that expedites such cases but can shield doctors from government regulators and the public."

When doctors are removed as defendants they are not reported to the National Practitioner Data Bank, a federal program that tracks malpractice payments and is used by the health care industry to do background checks on physicians. Neither are the doctors likely to be scrutinized by the Maryland Board of Physicians—not that many doctors shudder at that prospect.

Paul Bekman told Schulte that Hopkins has asked him to drop doctors as defendants. He said he is "more than willing" to agree, because doing so speeds up settlements. He cited the 2003 case of John Adrian, who went to Hopkins for a procedure to remedy acid reflux.

Hopkins surgeon Mark Talamani, walking alongside his patient as he was being wheeled into the operating room, mentioned, by-the-by, that he'd be using a new robotic device to do the procedure. Talamani didn't tell John Adrian that he had "limited experience" with the new gizmo.

The procedure to relieve indigestion wound up taking more than six hours, and in getting the hang of the robotic device, Talamani inadvertently cut a hole in Adrian's stomach.

Recuperating for more than a month and finally escaping with his life from Johns Hopkins critical care, Adrian sued both Hopkins and Talamani. Hopkins lawyers made it clear that this whole thing could be taken care of more quickly if Talamani were dropped from the suit, and it was done. Johns Hopkins settled and Talamani made a clean getaway.

After getting an eyeful of the Camden Yards outfield, I sat at Bekman's desk and began telling him what happened to Pam. He listened for a few minutes and then waived me off. "OK," he said, pulling a contract out of a drawer. "They hurt your wife. Let's get 'em. I get a third."

I liked that.

I signed, and he put the contract back in a drawer and the meeting was over.

I'd met with four lawyers about Pam's case. Each of them, including Bekman, told me that I should feel very fortunate about their willingness to accept the case because they only take a small percentage of the cases they are asked to handle. It's meant to make you feel special, but again, it's just business.

I'd seen so many ads for lawyers proclaiming their zeal to stick up for the underdog that I'd started to believe it. We did feel fortunate that Paul Bekman saw the merit of Pam's case and that he was going to go to bat for us.

But Walter v. Hopkins was just another cherry picked for the overflowing basket of Salsbury, Clements, Bekman, Marder & Adkins.

The firm dips its bread in the gravy rendered from the slam-dunk cases, the Josie Kings, with maximum return on negligible outlay.

Of course, an attorney is never going to turn down a promising case, no matter how backed up the office may be. Overworked grunts do the triage and worry about looming deadlines. (Bekman was often out on the lecture circuit, or appearing at law school forums with Rick Kidwell, his worthy opponent from Johns Hopkins, to discuss the purported malpractice crisis.)

I know of more than a few cases of medical malpractice victims being unable to find a lawyer because their case is too complicated and therefore too expensive to pursue, or the victim, though plainly mangled, was past the salad days, so recoverable lost income wasn't worth chasing.

"We'll be in touch," Bekman told me as I left.

This was good, I thought, because Pam had been declared to be disabled by the Social Security Administration as of March 25th, 2002—the date she entered Johns Hopkins Hospital and I'd had to run our business myself since then.

I was barely keeping up with our main store and the second store was now expensively languishing in a strip mall in another county. We were on the road to financial ruin.

I imagined that since Pam had the best lawyer in Baltimore who had a special relationship with Hopkins, he'd be able to wrap this whole thing up rather quickly. I imagined him poring over the records, building an ironclad case on the myriad of blunders that had occurred. He would then lay out the facts and present a withering case to Hopkins. He would demand satisfaction, and they would be eager to settle.

Six months later, with Pam still reeling from her ordeal and unable to help me keep our business afloat, I called Bekman to see how the plan was progressing, but I was told that he was out of the office and would call me back.

I waited a week and then called him again. His secretary said she would certainly make sure he got the message and that he would definitely call me back. Another week went by, and I called again. This time I got him. "Well," I said anxiously, "What's going on?" He told me that he was working on it and that we had to be patient and he said he would call back.

I fell into a pattern of calling him every two to three months. When I did catch him in, he always counseled patience. These things take time, he'd say.

Finally, two and a half years after our first meeting, I called Bekman and said I was coming up there and I was bringing Pam to his office so that she could finally meet him and we could discuss the case. We had a lot of questions. We wanted to know how and why this happened and we were eager to see what our lawyer had discovered.

He pulled a thin folder from his desk. "I've sent these records out to four cardiologists and none of them say that Hugh Calkins failed to deliver the standard of care."

Pam was livid. "The standard of care! Does that include me winding up in open-heart surgery?"

Bekman looked puzzled. "They didn't cut you, did they?"

Chapter 37

The Great Chest Tube Mystery

THEY CUT HER ALL RIGHT. They cracked open her chest the way a personal injury lawyer would crack open a lobster to celebrate a class action windfall. This case had been on Bekman's back burner for so long, he'd forgotten all about it. It's another business model: You take all the decent looking cases that come in the door, thereby depriving the competition of the business, and you really don't have to worry about them until the statute of limitations is suddenly looming.

The expert cardiologists who reviewed the records for Bekman were all Calkins chums from the Afib ablation club. Asking these docs to testify was laughable. Even if one were inclined to commit professional suicide by calling out a colleague, all he had to go on was a sanitized and exculpatory procedure report.

I would get all the records myself, and I would find out exactly what happened up there, and then I would get another lawyer.

It took me a while to figure out how hospitals deal with unruly patients. If you ask for records while your loved one is still in the hospital, they note that fact in the patient's chart, and they hunker down and start being very careful about what they say and what they write. Then once the patient is discharged and wheeled out the front door, or is rolled feet first out the back door, the victim's records are meted out to relatives as slowly as possible. It is part of the overall strategy of delay, to wear the enemy down, or just plain outlive them.

Thus my requests for Pam's complete medical record yielded meager results at first. I asked for a complete set of records in January of 2003. They sent what they said was the entire record, 302 pages, in August.

By 2005, I had them up to about 500 pages. Pam being a nurse, we knew with each delivery of the "entire record" that certain things were still missing. She was especially curious as to why there was a certain scar on the side of her chest. She knew it came from insertion of a chest tube, as for draining fluids or re-expanding a collapsed lung, but she could find no mention of it in the charts.

I contacted the Maryland State Attorney's office, which sent Hopkins a letter reminding them that there were, after all, rules about such things, and a patient was entitled to her records. That's when Hopkins coughed up 735 pages and an affidavit swearing up and down that that was everything. It was two years after my first request. But still, Pam could find nothing about a chest tube insertion. I told her that I thought the chest tube scar wasn't that important to the case. Let it go, I told her.

But Pam would not let it go.

We sent for records again, and a few months later a smiling FedEx man came to my door and handed me a box containing 742 pages. The new material included a three page document from Hugh Calkins labeled "Note to the Medical Chart." Dated May, 2002, it was written at the direction of Hopkins' in-house lawyer, a cranky guy named Rick Kidwell.

As per the protocol, Kidwell had been notified that someone was asking for medical records after some unpleasantness down in the EP Lab. He rang up Calkins to ask for a memo. This memo was to be written so as to cast the institution and its staff in a certain light regarding the affair.

And Calkins generally did a masterful job.

If the events had unfolded the way he described, there would be little room for complaint from patient Pam Walter; a malcontent, a sore loser who was upset at a bad outcome. But he made a couple of big mistakes that wound up defeating the purpose. Since the letter was meant to be a privileged communication between attorney and physician, it should have been addressed to Rick Kidwell and delivered to his office. But Calkins dictated the letter to his secretary as a note to the medical chart and had her fax a copy to Kidwell.

The letter was kept with Pam's records in his office, close to his vest, for four years. But when Pam asked for another copy of the entire chart out of the blue—and after the statute of limitations for a malpractice action had passed—someone in his office finally complied with the request.

So it happened that one day in July 2006, I sat cross-legged in a sea of papers in the middle of our living room floor, reading a very well done CYA memo. And at the very end of the memo Calkins writes this:

"I should note here that Dr. Richard Wu was manipulating the catheter at the time it became entrapped in the mitral valve."

This is the letter I was holding in my hand the day I got Richard Wu on the phone down at UT Southwest Medical Center, when he told me he was not involved in the *complication*.

I took the elevator to the 15th floor of the William Donald Schaefer Tower and handed a legal envelope to a clerk in the Maryland Health Claims Alternative Dispute Resolution Center. It was quarter to four on March 24th 2005. The three-year statute of limitations for Pam's malpractice case against Johns Hopkins would expire in an hour and forty-five minutes. Because we couldn't get a new lawyer so close to the deadline, we had to file the lawsuit ourselves, and then try to get a lawyer to take over.

The clerk took my check for the filing fee and time-stamped 4 copies of the twenty page complaint, which I'd printed out on my home computer a few hours earlier. She handed me my copy. "Hopkins, huh?" she said. "Watch out."

I laughed a little. I thought she was kidding.

Having had no legal training, our plan was simple and straightforward. We put all our cards on the table. Our whole case was clearly spelled out and documented in the complaint. In addition to standard language about negligence and causation, a solid case was made for a lack of informed consent, mostly quotes from Calkins himself describing the procedure as dangerous, unproven, unsafe and ineffective.

Hopkins had farmed the case out to Mairi Pat Maguire, a former RN, a nurse gone bad in my book by way of turning into a corporate defense lawyer, the two professions being at the very opposite of the spectrum for compassion, humanity and morals.

The case languished in the Health Claims Dispute Resolution Office for three years while Mairi Pat argued that it should be thrown out because we didn't have an expert witness. I was trying to find a lawyer all that time, but it turns out lawyers don't like Informed Consent cases or *Pro Se* cases.

Finally, we had to withdraw from arbitration and file the case in Circuit court, where it was summarily dismissed because we didn't have an expert witness.

But as I read the law, you didn't need an expert witness for an informed consent case to get into court, and once you got there, you could call the defendant doctor as your witness. I found a lawyer who agreed, and who filed and won an appeal.

Eight years after her trip to Hopkins, Pam would get her day in court.

Chapter 38

Hey, it could happen to anyone

WHEN HE'S OUT on the circuit, giving talks at various cardiology gatherings around the country, Calkins presents his findings—the results from the studies he performs on people— with the air of a storied combat vet at the local American Legion hall. "I learned a lot of things the hard way about the Lasso catheter," he tells colleagues. "One thing is you can Lasso a lot of things with it, including the mitral valve and if you happen to Lasso the mitral valve it's hard to untangle the valve. When we tried to untangle the valve we wound up ripping the valve and having to replace the valve, and I can tell you that was one memorable Lasso experience…"

Of course, even the most vivid memories can fade in the fog of litigation. The lawyer here might as well have been deposing the Magic 8-Ball: Did you tell Pam Walter that you did not know if the benefits of the procedure outweighed the risks?

Reply hazy, try again.

Nevertheless, thanks to court ordered depositions, we have a permanent and public record of how Richard Wu and Hugh Calkins recall the unfolding events of March 25, 2002—and on the subject of who was actually performing the procedure, Calkins puts forth fuzzy scenarios. Contrary to his customary "showing up to be there during the burn," as he confided to colleagues at an FDA hearing, on this particular day he *would have* scrubbed out after the procedure was set in motion, leaving the trainee at the wheel.

But he is insistent on the point that he was doing the critical part of the procedure. "I would de-scrub when it's time to analyze the figures to find out if the vein was isolated," Calkins said. "This isn't just looking at something. It's very tricky to do this."

"This is the critical part of the procedure. That's the part I was performing. That's what I was doing and then the catheter got entrapped."

He is trying to downplay the fact that he was not the primary operator for the procedure. That task had been delegated—without the patient's knowledge—to a trainee named Richard C. WU.

Repeat after me: "I was performing the most critical aspect of the procedure."

I can see a tense session in a conference room between Calkins and his lawyer just before his deposition. He's not used to being grilled and he's nervous.

"I was performing the most critical aspect of the procedure..."

Of course, it was Richard Wu who was the primary operator, and who was by definition performing the most critical aspect of the procedure. But Hopkins is very determined to keep Dr. Wu out of the picture. They do not want people to get the idea that they are running some kind of research mill up there and letting rookies pinch-hit for the big names that pull in the customers. It could be a money thing. Johns Hopkins Medicine is already listed in the Federal Contractor Misconduct Database for doing just that:

> "According to the allegations, Johns Hopkins submitted or caused the submission of false claims to the Medicare program on behalf of certain faculty physicians employed by the university without documentation to show that these physicians were personally involved in providing the services claimed by JHU. Instead, the government contends these services were actually delivered by an intern or resident of the teaching hospital."

Aside from defrauding the government, Hopkins is like other businesses in this way.

Johnny Cochran makes the pitch to you, but once you sign on the dotted line, lesser lights handle your case. There must be thousands and thousands of patients out there who underwent surgery at Johns Hopkins and to this day do not know who really did the job on them.

Defrauding the government is apparently another bedrock principle of the Hopkins business model.

In 2004, Hopkins Inc. agreed to pay $2.6 million for over billing the NIH for research projects from 1994 through 2000. The salaries of some Hopkins researchers and employees were being totally paid by the taxpayer—billed out to two or three government agencies at a time.

When you are trying to conceal facts, a deposition can be a real minefield. A big claymore for Calkins here is that under no circumstances can he allow himself to admit that the catheter was in the left ventricle of the heart:

So you were performing the critical part of the procedure on the other side of the room when the catheter got itself caught up in the mitral valve muscles. How exactly did it get there?

> "If you ask how is it possible for this catheter to get caught in the mitral valve, the answer is it is possible. It occurred. And you may ask, 'How can that possibly be?' And the answer is, One, the atrium is a small structure. And B, [*sic*] all the pulmonary veins are relatively close to the mitral valve. Three, we don't have our hands in the atrium. As a surgeon, we're working from the leg, we're four feet away.

> "So you have a small structure, the heart's beating, you have a catheter in the heart, the structures are all relatively close together, and obviously the mitral valve dipped back and caught on the catheter. One way or the other, we know for sure the Lasso catheter was stuck in the valve. So it happened."

This is perhaps the reason that Hugh Calkins is not a surgeon, despite his Freudian desires.

All of the experts—and quite a few laymen—stand solidly behind the principle that it's physically impossible for a heart valve to make a lunge for anything.

He's trying to conjure up a picture of a catheter tip snagging on the leaf of the valve. But this catheter had been fed into the ventricle through the valve, corkscrewing its way down through the working muscle strings until it hit bottom. The catheter was completely and ineluctably tangled in the mitral valve root at the base of the left ventricle—in the wrong chamber of the heart.

Did the catheter get caught in the mitral valve during repositioning to another site?

"It's hard to know if it was during the positioning, the repositioning or exactly when. What was the question? I don't know exactly when. I don't know how the catheter got caught in the valve. That is unknown to me. I know that it did. That's a fact. How it got caught, I don't know."

And who actually repositioned the catheter?

"I don't know for sure, but I suspect that it was Dr. Wu."

That was a pretty good hunch since Calkins wasn't even scrubbed in when Wu blundered into the wrong heart chamber.

And how did the catheter get so tangled in the muscles of the mitral valve that it ripped the muscles out of the heart when someone yanked on it?

"Okay. So the fact we know the mitral valve — the catheter got entangled on the mitral valve. What we don't know is how it happened. The possibilities are that the catheter, in order for the catheter to get trapped in the valve, the catheter had to be hitting the same location of the valve apparatus."

"So that could happen in one of two ways. Either the catheter moved toward the valve or the valve moved toward the catheter. If the question is how can the valve move toward the catheter... the valve can move posterior to the atrium."

These are not the ramblings of a Bellevue intern gone mad, these are the very considered thoughts of a graduate of Harvard Medical School.

And despite all the hemming and hawing and the dancing, Hugh Calkins knew exactly how the catheter got caught in my wife's mitral valve. He told his colleagues all about it that night at the Westin Copley Place hotel in Boston in 2006.

"The lawyers tell you, 'Well in the package instructions it says to never place the catheter near the mitral valve.' Well if you know where the pulmonary veins are, they are very near the mitral valve so it's very hard to not Lasso the valve occasionally..."

He was more specific when he wrote about it in 2007, two years before he swore truthfulness at a deposition: "Entrapment of the mitral valve apparatus by a mapping catheter results from inadvertent positioning of the catheter into the ventricle with counterclockwise rotation."

Richard Wu has a rich imagination.
"How many times, before Mrs. Walter, did you participate in a similar procedure in which you were the primary operator..."
"I know I did about 500 procedures..."
"How many where you were operating the catheter ..."
"I did somewhere between 250 to 300..."
"How many where you were the primary operator..."
"I think between 30 to 50..."
"With you as the primary operator? Is that what you're saying?"
"Less than 30."

I would point out here that ZERO qualifies as fewer than thirty, and that you or I or SpongeBob SquarePants could legitimately claim likewise. Mr. Wu does admit that he first laid eyes on Pam Walter on the morning of the procedure. "I have records stating that I wrote a history and a physical for Ms. Walter at 7am. on March 25th 2002," he said. He's not necessarily swearing to the facts, just to what the record states. By design, reality and the record are two different things.

Did you discuss the risks of the procedure with Pam Walter?

"Oh, yes. We went over the consent form before the procedure and we discussed the risks of the procedure. There on the consent form it lists pain and infection and bleeding, damage to blood vessels which may cause a blood clot or require surgical repair, nausea or vomiting from the sedation. The other things we discussed were perforation of the heart or lung which may require emergency intervention, respiratory risks that may require intervention, stroke, myocardial infarction or death ..."

He went on like that for a while.

Pam's daughter Kristi and I were with her at 7am in a patient receiving area. Pam was given a clipboard with forms to fill out and permissions to sign. I stayed with her until she was taken to the pre-op room, which was at 7:30 according to nurses' notes. Kristi went with her and stayed with her in the pre-op room until 8:10 when, according to the record, Pam was taken to Room One at the EP Lab. She was in the lab at 8:20 and by 8:27 she had been administered narcotic. None of us saw Wu or Calkins that morning.

And how long did it take Richard Wu to review the history, give her a physical examination and ensure that the informed consent process was faithfully discharged on the morning of the procedure?

"About a half hour," says Dr. Wu, under oath.

Chapter 39

A Vigorous Defense

> "Barracudas are elongated fish with prominent sharp-
> edged, fang-like teeth that are all of different sizes
> which are set in sockets of their large jaws. They have
> large pointed heads with an under bite in many species.
> Diamond rings and other shiny objects have been
> known to catch their attention."

> *-Wikipedia*

ENOUGH SAID.

You have to hand it to them. In court, my wife got crushed like an empty beer can. A lawyer friend told me that it made perfect sense for Johns Hopkins Medicine to have a woman lawyer defend this case, because only a woman could disembowel another woman on the stand and get away with it. He told me that, even among trial lawyers, women who do combat in courtrooms for corporate interests are notorious for having no scruples. "But," he said, "You can't hate them for it. They are doing their job."

I suppose. But it is deeply troubling to watch deliberate cruelty in action.

Chapter 40
The Operative Facts

ONCE THE TRIAL DATE was set, the Hopkins team set about, motion by motion, to dismantle Pam's case. The fact that it was, in effect, ghost surgery and that Richard Wu did the job instead of Hugh Calkins was dismissed as a cause of action. By the time the trial started only one count against Hopkins was left standing, which was this:

"... that Dr. Calkins did not inform Plaintiff that he (Dr. Calkins) did not know the safety and efficacy of the procedure, that he believed the procedure to be experimental... The operative facts required to prove the original claim involve what Dr. Calkins knew as of March 25, 2002, about the safety and efficacy of the procedure and Dr. Calkins' competency and skill level to perform the procedure on that date."

Which was OK with me, seeing as how there was plenty of proof that Hugh Calkins did not know whether the procedure was safe or effective, that he did indeed consider it to be experimental, and that he considered it to be very technically challenging to him–and that he failed to inform my wife of these facts.

It was the essence of the case, and his feelings about the very rough edges of the procedure were all over the Internet in articles and seminars he'd given over the years.

Then, on the morning the trial was supposed to begin, there came from the defense a great storm of Motions in Limine, motions on the threshold, and it took the judge so much time to go through these and grant each one that the trial was postponed two weeks. These were very unpleasant times for Pam and me. Her case was being whittled down to nothing; we were frustrated at every turn. The air conditioner broke on our car and there were some long hot rides home from Baltimore.

Still, there was hope. Pam would at least get to see Hugh Calkins get on the witness stand and explain himself. The jury would hear all those statements that he made.

Chapter 41

The Whole Truth

WITH THE JURY OUT OF the room, Pam and I were called to the bench. Hopkins' lawyers stood to our left, Pam's lawyer stood to our right.

The judge told my wife that when she took the stand to testify, she was not to refer to any aspect of the procedure. She was not to make any reference to her injuries. She was not to say anything about how she was injured. She was not to say anything about how a catheter got tangled in her mitral valve. She was not to say anything about who was operating the catheter when that happened.

Under no circumstances was she to refer to the procedure as being experimental or investigational. She was not to say anything about how Hugh Calkins described her as being "collateral damage."

She was not to say anything about having been in a coma or having suffered a stroke. She was not to say anything about her having to take blood thinners for the rest of her life or the fact that she has a prosthetic mitral valve. She was not to talk about how much this hurt her. She was not to talk about how much this cost her.

She was not to say anything about how any of this affected her.

Her eyes began to brim over with tears and she looked back at Hugh Calkins who was sitting at the defense table and she said,

"But he lied to me..." And she turned back to the Judge and she said "I can't say anything. Why are we even here?"

The Judge shrugged his shoulders.

All that she would be allowed to do would be to agree that she signed a consent form.

Pam did not get to see Hugh Calkins take an oath to tell the truth and then do just the opposite on the witness stand. Calkins testified earlier in the day, and we were late for court because Pam was up all night with severe abdominal cramps and was passing blood that morning—the effects of the blood thinners she has to take in order to stay alive.

Calkins testified under oath that I was not there with Pam when she twice visited him in his office prior to the procedure, or on the morning of the procedure—even though my signature is there as witness when she signed the generic consent form at 7am that day.

Chapter 42

Medicine, the Law and Common Decency

I STILL HAVE TROUBLE trying to understand the breathtaking cruelty that was inflicted on my wife in that Baltimore City courtroom in the first week of May 2010.

My wife is a kind, decent and generous person whose crime was to seek medical help at what is supposed to be one of the finest medical facilities in our country. Instead of getting care and compassion at Johns Hopkins, she was tricked, lied to, disfigured, maimed and mauled, and then tossed aside as collateral damage, a sacrifice to the career ambitions of Hugh G. Calkins, MD.

The legal profession took it from there, throwing every roadblock imaginable in her path as she sought simple justice.

When, after eight years of delay, she had finally gotten her day in court, Hopkins' defense lawyers launched an unrelenting and vicious assault. They put her on the stand and bullied and berated her for a full day, using legal tricks to force her to confirm the little slivers of misleading facts that were fed to the jury.

Forced to wait outside the courtroom, I could hear the muffled voice of Hopkins lawyer Mairi Pat Maguire as she mercilessly and relentlessly browbeat Pam on the first day, and I could glimpse, when the courtroom door would occasionally open, the sad, scared and tearful face of my wife as she struggled to withstand the assault.

That night, she woke at 2 AM with severe abdominal pain and was up all night, retching and writhing in pain and passing blood in the morning. I called the courthouse to let the judge's office know that she was terribly sick and might have to go to the hospital instead of the courtroom that day, but no quarter was given, so she returned to the witness stand that afternoon and the verbal beating was continued until she broke down on the stand and the jury had to be cleared from the room.

When she had cried herself out, the judge, giving no comfort or soothing words whatsoever, had the jury brought back in, and the thrashing continued. All the while Hugh Calkins sat observing, as he would a specimen stuck on a pin in his lab, as Pam struggled to get the truth out.

Still, she was brave and defiant, and I am proud of her because, for example, she would not agree — even after stern admonishments from the judge — that a heavily redacted consent form was a true document.

As the case was about to go to the jury, Hopkins made one last motion to dismiss. Without looking at or acknowledging Pam in any way, the judge told the jury that they were no longer needed, and then he smacked his gavel down and said this case is dismissed. The jury bolted gleefully like sixth graders at the last bell on the last day of school.

The judge bantered and joked with the gloating defense attorneys as he turned his back on us and left the bench.

We had lost.

Chapter 43
Epilogue

Read All About It!

> "I can't think of a procedure in the history of medicine where we've gone to patients and say this is very expensive, it's very dangerous, we have no idea what good it does you, but we'd like to do it, and if we can talk you into a trial we're just going to see how many of you have serious adverse events." – Dr. Doug A. Morrison

THE LEAD ARTICLE in the January, 2010 issue of the Journal of the American Medical Association, (Vol. 303, No.4) is about a study that found Afibbers would do much better to undergo catheter ablations instead of taking pills.

Usually you'd have to be a subscriber, or be willing to cough up $15 to read an article in JAMA. But the full text of *Comparison of Antiarrhythmic Drug Therapy and Radiofrequency Catheter Ablation in Patients with Paroxysmal Atrial Fibrillation: a Randomized Controlled Trial*, can be had on their site for free. It comes with a video presentation and a link to a patient information page. It's all courtesy of Biosense Webster, one of the Johnson & Johnson family of companies, the one that manufactures the NaviStar ThermoCool Irrigated Tip Catheter, the device vindicated in the study they sponsored.

The mainstream media basically reprinted Johnson & Johnson's press release, using headlines like this: Heart Procedure Beats Drugs for Irregular Heartbeat.

As they say in the PR business, this study had a big roll out. Many top names in the catheter ablation business had signed on: Natale, the best in the world at performing the procedure, and Pappone and Marchlinksi. And this was a vindication of sorts for Hugh Calkins, who'd been there from the very beginning, because the Navablator was really the latest evolution of the

REVELATION TX catheter system, for which he had gotten pilloried so long ago at the Holiday Inn.

The campaign to promote the news of this positive development for Johnson & Johnson's bottom line was enormously successful. The good word for Afib sufferers was spread far and wide with lots of radio and TV coverage: Catheter ablation for atrial fibrillation is here, and it works, and it is good for you. They made Google News and USA Today and The New York Times. They got the procedure performed live on the Today Show.

The PR effort was a real tour de force, and making the JAMA article free to the masses was a nice touch. Providing links to the article conveys openness, confidence and transparency, while actually supplying the opposite. The press release is written in plain English and outlines the methods of the study in general terms. But the reporter who looked past the press release at the JAMA article and the actual data was met with an undecipherable thicket of academic prose, beginning with the fact that this was a Bayesian-designed study and randomization sequences were generated by the sponsor statistician using SAS version 8.2 and stratified by site, with block sizes of 11 and 4...

How can you argue with that—especially when you're on deadline?

One senses the statistical sleight of hand in the aggressive number crunching, and I am told that a Bayesian method allows for cherry picking. In case you didn't know, Bayesian is a system for describing epistemological uncertainty using the mathematical language of probability.

Whatever that means, it seems certain to have enabled interested parties to make the swirling numbers come to rest in a particular pattern.

The pliable Bayesian system was suggested by AdvaMed, the Advanced Medical Technology Association, which exerts political muscle for the device manufacturers. "FDA should be open to the use of hybrid and/or Bayesian statistical analysis that allow pooling of already enrolled subject data with the new study design data, without inflicting a sample size penalty, or weighting one data set more than the other." Roughly translated, this means that the study should carry one of those tiny lines of print at the bottom of a diet pill commercial: "Results Not Typical"

For one thing, most people who suffer from atrial fibrillation were excluded from the study right off the bat. That's because people who have taken the drug amiodarone for their Afib were not allowed, and two thirds of Afib sufferers have been on amiodarone at one time or another. Amiodarone has its own drawbacks, but it is known to work better than ablation. "I don't think many people would argue that probably, head to head, amiodarone typically wins in trials," said Dr. Eric Prystowski at an FDA hearing on study methods.

Prystowski was a big booster for anti-arrhythmic drug therapy early on in the ablation vs. drugs debate. In 2005, while consulting for CV Therapeutics, a company that made pills instead of catheters, an interviewer wrote that "As for the argument that too many patients fail drug therapy and that it is ineffective long-term, Prystowski has longitudinal follow-up on patients in his practice for an average of six years, with some patients managed on drug therapy for more than 10 years. Overall, more than two thirds of his patients have remained in sinus rhythm, he said, noting that this follow-up is three or four years longer than any existing ablation follow-up."

Another muted aspect of the study was that the patients were relatively young, otherwise healthy people who suffered from paroxysmal bouts of Afib, and had their procedures done at hospitals with lots of experience. So the eye-catching headlines don't really apply to most people with the problem, who tend to be older people with more persistent atrial fibrillation.

Finally, Hugh Calkins, who nonetheless joined in the chorus of ablationists touting the study, pointed out the biggest flaw of all: The way the study was set up, there was no way that drug therapy could beat catheter ablation. The fix was in. Ablation was being compared to drug therapy in people who had already failed at drugs, and if you fail one drug, you're likely to fail a second. "What we're doing is sort of guaranteeing the drug arm's not going to work, you know, in virtually anyone," Calkins said to the FDA panel.

And he was not alone in his feelings. The FDA had been working on trial designs for the procedure since 1998, and the idea of comparing drugs to an invasive procedure for safety and effectiveness got shot down right away.

"We sought input from a significant number of electrophysiologists," said industry executive Burke Barett when the idea came up. "We were told by many of them that a study comparing A.F. ablation and medication did not make for strong clinical science because patients that failed a drug are being randomized to additional drug therapy as the control."

George Washington University's Dr. Cynthia Tracy, a consultant to the panel, said "To me, it doesn't make any sense to compare the risk of anti-arrhythmic drug therapy with the risk of catheter ablation... you are comparing apples and oranges. A patient is at a heck of a lot more risk on the day they are having their ablation done than on the day they are just taking amiodarone."

Dr. George Vetrovec from Virginia Commonwealth University had prescient objections. "I just don't want you stopping the drug and then ablating them and then starting the drug again and calling it a success," he said. "You see the problem; because you might just leave him on the amiodarone and you will never have another spell and you will credit it to ablation, and it really had nothing to do with that."

Dr. Tony Simmons from Wake forest University summed it up. "Trying to randomize them to drugs is just not going to work, right? We all agree to that. There is certainly enough historical data on drug therapy for atrial fibrillation to establish criteria on drug therapy, plus it is not a comparable control. So doing a randomized study comparing some ablation technique to drug therapy for atrial fibrillation is kind of a meaningless study."

Dr. Douglas Morrison told the panel that he didn't think much of the trial design--or of the whole concept of catheter ablation for atrial fibrillation. "It starts with a population of low risk, young people, no structural heart disease and predominantly paroxysmal atrial fibrillation. And to put it bluntly, as a non E.P. person, I'm just anxious to give you all enough rope to hang yourselves, because I think that it's very hard to demonstrate, even compared to beta blockers and calcium channel blockers, that ablation changes life very much. I can't think of a procedure in the history of medicine where we've gone to patients and say this is very expensive, it's very dangerous, we have no idea what good it does you, but we'd like to do it, and if we can talk you into a trial we're just going to see how many of you have serious adverse events..."

Speaking of adverse events, the JAMA article describes the Navablator experience this way:

"Catheter ablation was associated with a favorable safety profile in this study. Major adverse events have been reported in up to 6% of patients undergoing AF ablation, including thromboembolic events, atrialesophogeal fistula, cardiac perforation, phrenic nerve paralysis, and death. None of these more serious complications occurred in our study."

The J&J study protocol set acceptable risks for the Navablator at 7 percent. In fact, the actual rate of serious adverse events reported to the FDA in the study was 10.8%.

But that's OK says J&J, "The nature and types of adverse events experienced in this trial nonetheless represent an acceptable risk profile." And until my FOIA request gets processed, we'll have to take their word for it. In the summary that the company sent the FDA, they say that out of 139 people, 15 people suffered serious adverse events. They list five people as having vascular access problems, one person with pulmonary edema, one person with pericardial effusion, one person with pericarditis - and five people who were "hospitalized."

"Let's be clear," wrote Larry Husten, Editor of Cardiobrief, "There is no evidence in the literature to support the statement of an 85-90% success rate for catheter ablation of atrial fibrillation. To present this kind of statistic to the general public, many of whom may have atrial fibrillation, or may know someone who has atrial fibrillation, is completely irresponsible. Catheter ablation is emerging as an important therapeutic option for some patients with atrial fibrillation, and it is indeed an impressive medical advance, but it comes with a lot of caveats."

Hugh Calkins already knew that.

In 2007, with his patient recruitment piece still up on the Hopkins site, he wrote an opinion piece for the journal Nature, in which he recommended that catheter ablation for Afib should not be considered as a first line therapy. He begins by repeating what he told the FDA four years earlier, that "the true efficacy of Afib ablation remains unknown."

SENATORS CHUCK GRASSLEY AND HERB KOHL have put the fear of God and the United States Justice Department into the collective heart of the American medical drug and device industry, which is why the disclosure for the J&J study looks like this:

Funding/Support: This study was funded by Biosense Webster, who provided the catheters used.

Financial Disclosures: Dr Wilber reported receiving grants fromBiosense Webster, Boston Scientific, Medtronic, and St Jude Medical; consulting fees from Biosense Webster, Medtronic, and Sanofi-Aventis; honoraria from Biosense Webster, Boston Scientific, Medtronic, and St Jude Medical; and royalties from Blackwell/Futura. Dr Pappone reported receiving grants and consulting fees from St Jude Medical and Johnson & Johnson, and honorarium from Biosense Webster. Dr Neuzil reported receiving grants from Biosense Webster, Cardiofocus, Cyrocath Technologies, Hansen Medical, NIH BARI 2D, and St Jude Medical; consulting fees from Stereotaxis; and honorarium from Biosense Webster. Dr De Paola reported receiving a grant from Bristol-Myers Squibb. Dr Marchlinski reported receiving grants and honoraria from Biosense Webster, Boston Scientific, and St Jude Medical; consulting fees from Biosense Webster, Boston Scientific, GE Healthcare, Medtronic, and St Jude Medical; and speakers' bureau fees from Biosense Webster. Dr Natale reported receiving grants from Biosense Webster and St Jude Medical, and speakers' bureau fees from Biosense Webster, Boston Scientific, Medtronic, and St Jude Medical. Dr Macle reported receiving consulting fees and honorarium from Biosense Webster. Dr Daoud reported receiving consulting fees from BARD and Biosense

Webster, and honorarium from Biosense Webster. Dr Calkins reported receiving consulting fees from Ablation Frontiers, Atricure, BARD, Biosense Webster, Boston Scientific, CryoCor, CyberHeart, Medtronic, ProRhythm, Sanofi-Aventis, and TASER International; a grant and honorarium from Biosense Webster; speakers' bureau fees from Atricure, BARD, Biosense Webster, Boston Scientific, Medtronic, and Reliant; and fellowship fees from BARD, Boston Scientific, and Medtronic. Dr Hall reported receiving consulting fees from Biosense Webster. Dr Reddy reported receiving grants from Atritech, Boston Scientific, Biosense Webster, Cardiofocus, CryoCath Technologies, Endosense Hansen Medical, St Jude Medical, and Stereotaxis; consulting fees from Biosense Webster and St Jude Medical; and honoraria from Boston Scientific, Biosense Webster, Medtronic, and St Jude Medical. Dr Augello reported receiving honoraria from BARD, Biosense Webster, and St Jude Medical. Dr Reynolds reported receiving consulting fees from Biosense Webster, Cardiome Pharma Corp, and Sanofi-Aventis. Mr Vinekar and Ms Liu are employees of Biosense Webster. Drs S. Berry and D. Berry reported receiving consulting fees from Biosense Webster, Veridex LLC, Boston Scientific, Endologix, R.R. Bard, W.L. Gore, Medtronic, Bristol-Myers Squibb, Pfizer, and Teva Pharmaceuticals.

The End

Post script:

The January, 2011 issue of The Journal of the American College of Cardiology carries a paper by Michele Haïssaguerre which reports the latest study results for catheter ablation for atrial fibrillation.

At a five-year follow up, the procedure had a 29% success rate, and the authors noted that "results in the real world may be even worse than those reported in the study…"

Hugh Calkins called these long-term results "sobering," considering that the investigators performing the ablation procedures are part of the group who pioneered the therapy.

J Am Coll Cardiol, 2011; 57:160-166, doi:10.1016/j.jacc.2010.05.061

SOURCE NOTES

Introduction

Rick Kidwell "... it's like the theory of sharks being attracted to blood in the water": JUH Magazine, June 1999, http://www.jhu.edu/jhumag/0699web/oncampus.html

A Mitral valve, Flapping in the Breeze, Prolapsed into the Atrium...

"Doctors love to patronize and dominate...": Issues in Medical Ethics *Volume 8, Number 4, October-December 2000*

"the attending shows up to be there during the burn.": Transcript, FDA Circulatory Systems Devices Panel meeting May 29, 2003
out selling TASER guns ... : PoliceOne.com, February 11, 2005, http://www.policeone.com/police-products/press-releases/99272/
one of the more common date rape drugs: Wikipedia http://en.wikipedia.org/wiki/Sedative

VERITAS

"The fact that this procedure was performed at a teaching hospital is not relevant..." Ward Ethics, Kushner, Thomasma, Cambridge University Press, 2001 The Responsibility of Informing, p 23

He was experimenting with two new ablation techniques and testing out a couple of new mapping catheters...: Transcript, Ablation Strategies for Management of Atrial Fibrillation, Lecture with Slides Hugh Calkins, MD
http://www.vindicomeded.com/cmelc/tc_lecture.asp?rid=17208

The Procedure: "Ready for Prime Time"

Study Affirms Value of Non-Surgical Treatment for Arrhythmia: JHMI Press Release, Jan 9, 1999,
http://esgweb1.nts.jhu.edu/press/1999/JANUARY1/990119.HTM;
JHMI Newsfeed, 1999,
http://www.hopkinsmedicine.org/hnf/hnf_951.htm
Finally a Way to get Rid of Afib: JHMI Press Release
http://www.hopkinsmedicine.org/hmn/W03/medrounds.cfm
heart*wire,* August 31, 2005,
http://www.theheart.org/article/546039.do

"Delay Would be Dangerous, Potentially Catastrophic"

Professor Luceri, who would later join Hugh Calkins... : Canadian Medical Association Journal CMAJ August 12, 2008; 179 (4). doi:10.1503/cmaj.1080079.
http://www.cmaj.ca/cgi/content/full/179/4/342-b

Progress continues in the quest to cure atrial fibrillation with catheter ablation techniques...": Eur Heart J (2001) 22(22): 2038-2040 doi:10.1053/euhj.2001.2757 H. Calkins
http://eurheartj.oxfordjournals.org/content/22/22/2038.full.pdf+html

The Cat's out of the Bag
Cynthia Tracy, Transcript, Circulatory System Devices Panel, V2, July 22, 1998, p118
http://www.fda.gov/OHRMS/DOCKETS/AC/98/transcpt/3442t2a.pdf

"Just because we can doesn't mean we should...":
Transcript, Circulatory System Devices Panel, V2, July 22, 1998, ibid p118
Vetrovec *I'll tell you how...* ibid p 188
A New System for Catheter Ablation ...:
A New System for Catheter Ablation of Atrial Fibrillation
American Journal of Cardiology Pages 227-236, 11 March 1999
http://www.ajconline.org/issues?issue_key=S0002-9149(00)X0105-1

The Bottom Line
Professor Calkins, consultant..: JAMA. 2010;303(4):333-340. doi:10.1001/jama.2009.2029
http://jama.ama-assn.org/cgi/content/full/303/4/333#AUTHINFO
TASER SEC Lawsuit ...:
http://www.glancylaw.com/pdf/TASER.pdf%20
More than 330 people haved died after being TASERed...:
http://www.amnesty.org/en/news-and-updates/report/tasers-potentially-lethal-and-easy-abuse-20081216
Death by TASER Dziekanski Taser YouTube Canada:
http://www.youtube.com/watch?v=05vuY-kqp9o
That was enough for Canadians...: TASERS in Medicine
http://ecmaj.ca/cgi/content/full/178/11/1401

The Alive or Dead Thing
Chilli catheter approval...:
http://www.accessdata.fda.gov/cdrh_docs/pdf/P980003a.pdf

Assets Calkins...: http://67.192.184.241/assets/files/calkins-prospective-comparision-of-lesions.pdf
Cardima Revelation Dog Studies
http://67.192.184.241/assets/files/calkins-prospective-comparision-of-lesions.pdf
Chilli ablation study:...: Catheter Ablation of Ventricular Tachycardia in Patients With Structural Heart Disease Using Cooled Radiofrequency Energy...: Journal of the American College of Cardiology
Volume 35, Issue 7, June 2000, Pages 1905-1914
Learning by Burning...: MARCHLINSKI, FRANCIS E. Insights into the Electrophysiology of Ventricular Tachycardia Gained by the Catheter Ablation Experience: Journal of Cardiovascular Electrophysiology 1994,Vol.5 DO - 10.1111/j.1540-8167.1994.tb01126.x http://dx.doi.org/10.1111/j.1540-8167.1994.tb01126.x

And Yes I said Yes I Will Yes
A perfunctory signing of a consent form..: http://www.forensic-psych.com/articles/artMedicalNegligence.php

A Dangerous Instrument
"We are missing a lot of things at this point ..." heart*wire, August 2005* http://www.theheart.org/article/546039.do

Presentations, Papers and Posters
Competition for technology...: Ethical Issues for Invasive Cardiologists:*Catheterization and Cardiovascular Interventions* Volume 61, Issue 2, pages 157–162, February 2004
http://onlinelibrary.wiley.com/doi/10.1002/ccd.v61:2/issuetoc
A hot night in Dixie...: (1998, November 12). Cardima Holds Annual Arrhythmia Symposium and Launches New Website at American Heart Association Meeting in Dallas *The Free Library*. (1998). Retrieved November 29, 2010 from http://www.thefreelibrary.com/Cardima Holds Annual Arrhythmia Symposium and Launches New Website at...-a053207967

Berger Pathfinder...:(1998, April 3). Cardima Successfully Treats First Patient in United States Atrial Fibrillation Study at the Johns Hopkins Hospital *The Free Library*. (1998). Retrieved November 29, 2010 from http://www.thefreelibrary.com/Cardima Successfully Treats First Patient in United States Atrial...-a020454690

Cardima... his company just posted a first quarter loss of nearly $4 million...: (2001, February 7). Cardima Announces Fourth Quarter and Full-Year Financial Results; Monthly Burn Rate Cut to Approximately $600,000 as Company Focuses on Phase III Clinical Trial for Atrial Fibrillation *The Free Library*. (2001). Retrieved November 29, 2010 from http://www.thefreelibrary.com/Cardima Announces Fourth Quarter and Full-Year Financial Results;...-a071123814

Breakthrough

Haïsseguerre *"Electrophysiological Breakthroughs From the Left Atrium to the Pulmonary Veins"* Circulation. 2000 Nov 14;102(20):2463-5.

Calkins "...he himself had all but abandoned the idea. Citing data from 1998": Calkins, a Practical Approach to Catheter Ablation for Atrial Fibrillation , Lippincott Williams & Wilkins, 2008

PR Newswire, "Patient was a 68 year old female … ": Cardima pres release, http://www.accessmylibrary.com/coms2/summary_0286-28402192_ITM

"the doctor put the catheder in my groin ..": http://forums.wrongdiagnosis.com/showthread.php?t=8584

"One can easily see how this can increase the number of approvals...": Kelpinski Robert J. Klepinski, Journal of Medical Device Regulation, 2009, 6 (2), 8-19 http://www.fredlaw.com/bios/attorneys/klepinskirobert/Klepinski_JMDRMay2009.pdf

Ochoa was the company's Regulatory Affairs Specialist who worked to get Haïsseguerre 's new Lasso catheter...: Lasso 510k

Approval
http://www.accessdata.fda.gov/cdrh_docs/pdf/K002333.pdf
FDA 510k letter: The "standard Cordis Webster Diagnostic 7F
Deflectable Catheter."
http://www.accessdata.fda.gov/cdrh_docs/pdf/K953663.pdf
Drawing, Webster Catheter United States Patent US4960134:
http://www.freepatentsonline.com/4960134.pdf
" doctors at Harvard would publish a paper" about Lasso catheter
entrapment : http://www.ncbi.nlm.nih.gov/pubmed/15851219

"Do We Know What We're Doing?"
Calkins: "I think all of us are aware of the fact that the published
literature probably tremendously overestimates the true efficacy of
catheter ablation…" http://tinyurl.com/CalkinsFDAProRhythm
"A typical case is someone who had pulmonary vein ablation
shows up in the ER...": Transcript, Ablation Strategies for
Management of Atrial Fibrillation, Lecture with Slides
Hugh Calkins, MD
http://www.vindicomeded.com/cmelc/tc_lecture.asp?rid=17208
"Just another risk to put on the consent form," ibid

"In some ways, EPs are operating blind... ":
http://www.theheart.org/article/116103.do
Calkins, Xray radiation Burns
http://onlinelibrary.wiley.com/doi/10.1111/j.1540-
8159.1997.tb03574.x/abstract
"Visualization of the catheter tip in relation to the cardiac anatomy
is crucial.": Medical Clinics of North America. P476 Vol 85 No. 2,
March 2001
"The Arrival of AFIB Ablation":
http://www.jhintl.net/forphysicians/default.aspx?id=3334
"but he has more sobering news …"
http://www.cardiosource.com/expertopinions/hottopics/article.asp?
paperID=228
""The true efficacy of Afib ablation remains unknown.": Nature
Reviews Cardiology 4, 4-5 (January 2007)
doi:10.1038/ncpcardio0741

http://www.nature.com/nrcardio/journal/v4/n1/full/ncpcardio0741.html

"Calkins went on to say" ...

http://www.medicalnewstoday.com/medicalnews.php?newsid=50308

The Ideal Candidate

"There are many areas in which there can be a conflict between the patient's best interest and the physician's own personal interest.... Calkins: "catheter ablation of AF should be considered to be an experimental procedure.": of Cardiac Arrhythmias Cardiology in Review: May/June 2001 - Volume 9 - Issue 3 - pp 121-130, http://journals.lww.com/cardiologyinreview/toc/2001/05000

Room for Improvement

"In this study, we provide analysis of AF ablation complications for 641 consecutive procedures. ": Journal of Cardiovascular Electrophysiology, Vol. 19, Issue 6, pp 627–631, June 2008.DOI: 10.1111/j.1540-8167.2008.01181.x http://onlinelibrary.wiley.com/doi/10.1111/j.1540-8167.2008.01181.x/full

"Patients were enrolled prospectively in a longitudinal patient database... ": ibid

Dr. Marcus Wharton at the Medical University if South Carolina posed a question...: Current Controlled Trials in Cardiovascular Medicine 1468-6708 2001 2 2 67 70 http://cvm.controlled-trials.com/content/2/2/067 10.1186/cvm-2-2-067 11806775 6 3 2001 13 3 2001 5 4 2001 2001 BioMed Central Ltd ablation atrial fibrillation pulmonary veins

A Dangerous Instrument

Around the time that Pam became one of the first 100 unwitting participants...: Hindricks Kottkamp: * Potential Benefits Risks and Complications of Catheter Ablation for Atrial Fibrillation, More Questions than Answers. Published August 2002 *Hindricks, Kottkamp*

J Cardiovasc Electrophysiol, Vol. 13, pp. 768-769, August 2002 :
http://www3.interscience.wiley.com/cgi-bin/fulltext/118959025/PDFSTART

It's Making Money for the Hospital
Gallagher, Gorden Tomassoni,and "Sonny" Jackman were interviewed about a catheter navigation system on the board at Stereotaxis: heart*wire*
http://www.theheart.org/article/116103/cite.do

Dr. Jackman serves as a paid consultant to Webster Laboratories, the manufacturer of the catheters used for ablation in this study....
N Engl J Med 1992; 327:313-318
http://prod.nejm.org/doi/full/10.1056/NEJM199207303270504#t=articleTop

Just One of Those Things
Johns Hopkins University President William R. Brody decided that he wanted JHU to get a piece of the action. (Baltimore) Daily Record, March 17, 2006
http://findarticles.com/p/articles/mi_qn4183/is_20060317/ai_n16143147/
The inspection turned up a number a irregularities and violations:
http://www.circare.org/fdawls2/stimsoft_20031027.pdf

The Spin You Put on It
"The process of obtaining informed consent from patients mandates..." Roderick Tung J Am Coll Cardiol, 2008; 52:1111-1121, doi:10.1016/j.jacc.2008.05.058
"the safety and efficacy of pulmonary vein ablation was unknown then [in 2000] and it is unknown now..
http://www.fda.gov/ohrms/dockets/ac/03/transcripts/3954t1.htm

How important is it for doctors to be careful with study data?
http://content.onlinejacc.org/cgi/content/full/52/14/1111

"I had an ablation over 3 months ago ...."
http://www.medhelp.org/posts/Heart-Disease/Chest-pain-following-ablation/show/10257

A Drink of Water
A Remedy of Errors:
http://www.hopkinsmedicine.org/hmn/S04/feature1.cfm
a rare display of pique by the FDA... :
http://www.fda.gov/ora/frequent/483s/JohnHopkins483.html
The FDA cited lack of informed consent... :
http://www.fda.gov/downloads/AboutFDA/CentersOffices/ORA/ORAElectronicReadingRoom/UCM064075.pdf

Two Months Later
"Serious underlying problems that could compromise the quality of mammography performed at your facility, they represent a violation of the law":
http://www.fda.gov/downloads/ICECI/EnforcementActions/WarningLetters/2001/UCM078215.pdf

another study that was even more similar to Tuskegee...:
Investigators' Responsibilities for Human Subjects in Developing Countries, Angell, Marcia , N Engl J Med 2000; 342:967-969, March 30, 2000 http://www.nejm.org/toc/nejm/342/13/
"Johns Hopkins Admits Scientist used Indian Patients as Guinea Pigs" British Medical Journal, Nov. 2001
http://www.circare.org/im/im13Aug2002.htm

The Gravy Train
Letter from the Food and Drug Administration regarding unregulated human experimentation...:
http://www.circare.org/bna05072003.pdf
The Baltimore Sun's Tom Pelton wrote about voluntary oversight...: http://www.uiowa.edu/cyberlaw/hsr/hsrepilo.html
"The February 2002 issue of JHU Magazine:
http://www.jhu.edu/jhumag/0202web/trials.html

introducing a bill that would shed some light on the whole human research situation...:http://mlis.state.md.us/2002rs/billfile/hb0917.htm
Physics Today reported in 2009 that Johns Hopkins University was the biggest recipient of US R&D funds...:http://physicstoday.org/
"It was a good thing for Hopkins, Inc...": M. Alexander Otto BNA's Medical Research Law & Policy Report, May 7, 2003 http://www.circare.org/bna05072003.pdf
Hopkins vice president Joanne Pollak told the Baltimore Sun: http://articles.baltimoresun.com/2002-03-15/news/0203150291_1_johns-hopkins-hopkins-medicine-research

Fine Wood Furniture
But he was a hard man to get a hold of, and an article in The American Medical News... http://www.ama-assn.org/amednews/2003/09/15/prsc0915.htm
"The council's rebuke had no impact. Johns Hopkins Magazine dutifully reported that "Nine days into ...": http://www.jhu.edu/jhumag/1103web/wholly.html
Johns Hopkins Penalized for Resident Hour Violations http://www.ama-assn.org/amednews/2003/09/15/prsc0915.htm

Patient Combative
"Most critical care nurses are familiar with the term ICU psychosis,": Brenda Hixon-Vermillion of the Ohio State University Medical Center, Nurseweek/Nursing Spectrum April 12, 2002 http://news.nurse.com/apps/pbcs.dll/article? AID=2002204120307

Not the Answer
"So really where I became enamored with Afib ablation..": Transcript, Ablation Strategies for Management of Atrial

Fibrillation, Lecture with Slides Hugh Calkins, MD
http://www.vindicomeded.com/cmelc/tc_lecture.asp?rid=17208

Hey, it Could Happen to Anyone
"I would de-scrub when it's time to analyze the
figures..":Deposition, Hugh Calkins, Pam Walter v. Hugh Calkins,
Johns Hopkins
"Johns Hopkins Medicine is already listed in the Federal
Contractor Misconduct
Database...":http://oig.hhs.gov/publications/docs/press/2003/02140
3release.pdf

Read All About It
"I can't think of a procedure in the history of medicine...": Dr.
Doug A. Morrison, Yakima, WA Heart Center, Transcript, p175
FDA Circulatory Systems Device Advisory Panel, Sept. 20, 2007
http://www.fda.gov/OHRMS/DOCKETS/ac/07/transcripts/2007-
4318t2-02.pdf
The lead article in the January, 2010 issue of the Journal of the
American Medical Association, (Vol. 303, No.4) http://jama.ama-
assn.org/cgi/content/full/303/4/333
Larry Husten "Let's be clear,":
http://www.kevinmd.com/blog/2010/02/treating-atrial-fibrillation-
catheter-ablation-tv-ethical.html

www.ingramcontent.com/pod-product-compliance
Lightning Source LLC
Chambersburg PA
CBHW072043280526
45788CB00006B/2161

* 9 7 8 1 4 5 6 4 7 1 6 0 6 *